HEALING IN ORDER

Why Chronic Illness Persists—and the Missing Sequence Behind Lasting Recovery

MARCUS ETTINGER, DC

Readers are invited to visit www.thebookhealinginorder.com for updates on the research in this book, additional educational resources, and ongoing developments in the Ettinger Foundation Protocol (EFP) framework.

Healing in Order
Why Chronic Illness Persists—and the Missing Sequence Behind Lasting Recovery

Marcus Ettinger, DC

Hardcover ISBN 979-8-9975134-1-2
Paperback ISBN 979-8-9975134-2-9

The Ettinger Foundation Protocol (EFP), including its terminology, framework, phases, and methodology as presented in this book, is an educational framework developed by the author. It is intended to facilitate understanding of physiologic healing and is not a substitute for individualized medical diagnosis or treatment.
See the full Disclaimer on the following page.

1. Disclaimer

Healing in Order is intended for educational and informational purposes only. The information presented in this book is designed to help readers better understand the physiologic principles that influence healing and recovery. It is not intended to provide individualized medical advice, diagnosis, or treatment, nor does reading this book establish a doctor-patient relationship with the author.

Healing and illness are highly individual. The physiologic concepts discussed in this book should not be interpreted as recommendations for the diagnosis or treatment of any specific medical condition. Every person's medical history, medications, health status, and treatment needs are unique. Readers should consult an appropriately qualified healthcare professional before making significant changes to their medical care, medications, supplements, diet, exercise program, or other health-related practices.

2. Foundation Work

The Foundation Work exercises included throughout this book are educational exercises designed to help readers apply the physiologic principles discussed in each chapter. They are intended to encourage habits and practices that may support the body's normal healing processes and overall health.

These exercises are not individualized medical advice, prescribed treatment, or a substitute for professional medical care. While many readers may find them helpful, they should not be interpreted as guarantees of benefit or as appropriate for every individual or every medical condition. The decision to implement any health-related practice should be made in consultation with an appropriately qualified healthcare professional who is familiar with your individual circumstances.

3. Scientific Understanding

Our understanding of human physiology continues to evolve. The concepts presented in this book are based on the scientific literature, established physiologic principles, and the author's clinical experience at the time of publication. As scientific knowledge advances, recommendations and interpretations may change.

Medicine and science are continually developing disciplines. No single book can account for every individual circumstance, every emerging discovery, or every possible clinical presentation.

4. Individual Results

The patient stories, examples, and clinical experiences described throughout this book are presented for educational purposes to illustrate physiologic principles. Identifying details have been changed, and in some cases characteristics have been combined to protect privacy.

These examples should not be interpreted as predictions, guarantees, or assurances that another individual will experience similar results. Recovery is influenced by numerous biological, environmental, genetic, and lifestyle factors that differ from person to person.

5. Personal Responsibility

The purpose of *Healing in Order* is to provide a framework for understanding how the body heals and why the sequence in which physiologic systems recover matters. Readers remain responsible for the healthcare decisions they make and should seek appropriate medical evaluation for any new, persistent, worsening, or concerning symptoms.

If you believe you are experiencing a medical emergency, seek immediate medical attention or contact your local emergency services.

To my wife,
You have allowed us to go on a twenty-three-year-long journey.
Sometimes with a map, sometimes with just an idea of where
I think we should go, uncovering the path along the way.

There have been triumphs as well as setbacks, but no setback
has ever stopped our forward progress for long.

You are my compass and my light.
You are the one constant in my life.
I love you.

To my close friends and family,
who have always been there.
You are the gold.

Table of Contents

Healing In Order Introduction: Before We Begin

by Marcus Ettinger, DC

I want to tell you something that took me a long time to be able to say plainly.

I have spent close to four decades in clinical practice. I have worked with thousands of patients across the full spectrum of chronic illness—fatigue syndromes, autoimmune conditions, post-viral recovery, digestive disorders, hormonal disruption, and multi-system dysfunction that resists a single diagnostic category. I have read the research, attended conferences and seminars, revised my thinking more times than I can count, and developed a clinical framework that now guides every case I see.

And for the first fifteen years of my practice, I made the same mistake most practitioners make, in one form or another, with patients who did not respond the way the evidence said they should.

I treated the problem I could see.

Not the wrong problem, necessarily. The right diagnosis. The right mechanism. The right treatment.

I just kept applying it in the wrong order.

And for years, I explained the failures away—the patient had an unusual sensitivity, the case was especially complex, or we simply had not yet found the correct approach. It took me longer than I would like to admit to recognize that I was not looking at a collection of unusual cases. I was looking at a consistent pattern.

And the pattern was telling me something I had not been trained to see.

The body does not heal in the order we choose.

It heals in the order it requires.

The patients who taught me this were not dramatic cases. They were people who had done everything right.

They had seen competent practitioners. They had followed thoughtful recommendations. They had been compliant, patient, informed, and determined. They had tried the things that should have worked and had not given up when those things failed.

Many arrived with binders, with timelines, and with the exhaustion of a person who has spent years trying to solve a problem that keeps changing shape.

And many of them, without being able to articulate it precisely, had arrived at the same suspicion: that something in their body was fundamentally broken. That they were uniquely resistant to healing. That the trajectory of their life was going to be organized, from this point forward, around the management of an illness that could not truly be resolved.

Many had stopped arguing against the suspicion. They had simply begun, slowly, to build their lives around it.

That suspicion was wrong.

What was broken was not the body.

What was broken was the sequence.

This book is built around a simple idea: the body recovers from chronic illness in a biologic order. Not the order of the loudest symptom or the most alarming lab finding, but the order required by the body's own regulatory architecture.

Each layer of recovery depends on the stability of the one beneath it.

Some systems cannot recover until the systems beneath them become stable enough to support recovery. A body living in protection cannot consistently invest in repair. A system overwhelmed by inflammation often cannot sustain deeper restoration. And a person can sleep for seven hours a night while still waking up physiologically unrecovered.

The sequence matters because recovery is layered and interconnected.

The sequence is not arbitrary. It reflects biological dependency.

And when treatment is aimed above the body's current recovery capacity, the treatment often fails to hold. In already-overloaded systems, it can make things worse. Not because the treatment itself is wrong, but because the conditions required for the body to absorb it have not yet been established.

This pattern appears across diagnostic categories, across symptoms, across specialties, and across patients whose illnesses look completely different from the outside.

Once you begin to recognize it, it becomes difficult not to see.

I want to speak to two people at once because both may be reading this book.

The first is the person who is ill.

Who has accumulated treatments that did not hold, improvements that collapsed, practitioners who were competent and caring, and still could not explain why the expected outcomes kept not arriving.

Who has gradually stopped trusting the predictability of their own body, started organizing life around uncertainty, and begun wondering whether the life they planned is still available to them.

If that is you, I want you to understand something before you read another page:

Your body is not behaving randomly.

What appears chaotic often has an underlying physiologic logic that becomes visible once the sequence is understood.

The treatment that made you worse was not proof that you were beyond help. The plateau that would not move was not necessarily failure, and the exhaustion of trying things that should have worked is not evidence that your body is uniquely resistant to healing.

The second person is the practitioner.

The physician, naturopath, chiropractor, functional medicine clinician, nurse practitioner, or health coach who has sat across from patients like those in this book and has felt, with increasing intensity, the frustration of doing everything the evidence supports and watching patients not improve.

I have sat in that position.

What I want to say to you is this:

The judgment is often sound.

The treatments are often correct.

What is frequently missing is not knowledge of what to treat, but recognition of when the body is capable of receiving the treatment being offered.

That is the problem this book attempts to clarify.

Throughout this book you will meet a group of composite patients whose lives illustrate these patterns. Their stories are drawn from years of clinical observation, and they are true in the way that matters most: they reflect what actually happens, again and again, in understandable and predictable ways.

Claire arrived with a three-inch binder and a section at the back labeled "Things That Made Me Worse." That section was the longest one.

David ran four mornings a week and had the blood panels to prove he was doing everything right, yet felt as though his body had stopped responding to the things that had once worked predictably.

Elena had five diagnoses and, as she put it, nobody had the box—the image on the front of the puzzle.

Rachel moved through the world as though her body no longer fully believed it was safe.

Thomas slept through the night and still woke feeling unrecovered.

Nadia knew exactly what rebuilding should produce and could not understand why it kept failing her.

These are not exceptional cases. They are representative ones.

This book will not tell you what to take. It will not give you a supplement protocol, a treatment plan, or a diagnosis. That is not something a book can responsibly provide—because the right treatment depends entirely on where you are in the recovery hierarchy, and that requires clinical assessment, not reading.

What this book will give you is something more durable: a framework for understanding how recovery actually works, and why the sequence matters as much as the specific treatment.

With that framework, you will be better equipped to understand your own history of illness, evaluate the approaches you have tried or been offered, and have more productive conversations with the practitioners you work with.

It will also give you something concrete to do.

At each layer of the hierarchy, there are foundational practices—specific ways of using light, breath, movement, food timing, and sleep—that are safe, accessible, and grounded in the same physiologic principles that guide the clinical framework itself.

The practices are ordinary. The sequence is what changes their effect.

Somewhere in the middle of this book, you may have a moment of recognition. Not a dramatic one, but quiet, the way real recognition is usually received.

A passage that describes something you have been experiencing for years and have never seen described precisely.

A line that explains something that has never been explained.

A patient story that feels, uncomfortably and then reassuringly, familiar.

That recognition is not incidental. It is the point.

The body's most frightening behaviors become less frightening once their logic becomes visible.

The treatment that made you sicker was not evidence that you were beyond help.

The plateau that would not move was not a permanent ceiling.

The crash that followed a period of progress was not proof that recovery was impossible.

These were physiologically coherent responses to conditions that had not yet been addressed in the order the body required.

Once you understand the sequence, the history changes its meaning.

Not what it cost, but what it was trying to tell you.

And meaning, it turns out, is not a small thing. The absence of an organizing explanation for suffering is itself a form of suffering, and this book is an attempt to provide that explanation.

Not to minimize what chronic illness costs or to offer false reassurance, but to give the history a logic it may never have had, and to offer the body the conditions—in the right order—under which it already knows how to heal.

The book is organized in the order the body requires.

We begin at the foundation and work upward through each layer of the hierarchy before moving into the chapters on regression, maintenance, and what recovery actually looks like once it arrives.

At each phase, we will meet patients whose experiences make the physiology recognizable. We will examine what that layer requires from the one beneath it, what it makes possible for the one above it, and what happens when treatment is aimed above a system's current recovery capacity.

One note before we begin.

This book was written for people living with chronic illness. But the patients I see with the pattern this book describes increasingly include people who became ill—or whose existing illness became significantly more complex—after a viral infection.

The sequence of recovery remains the same.

What changes is often the depth of the disruption and the patience the timeline requires.

You will meet Claire in the first chapter.

Claire made a full recovery.

It took nearly two years and demanded a level of patience she was not sure she possessed.

But this was real recovery—not merely managed, compensated, or maintained through ongoing treatments.

It was the kind of healing that eventually allowed her to stop thinking about her body and simply live inside it again.

She went back to the office, took the trip with her daughter, and made plans and kept them.

What recovery looked like, in practice, was not dramatic.

It was the absence of the calculation.

She made a dinner reservation without first mapping the exit.

She said yes to things without consulting an internal ledger of energy reserves.

She had a difficult week and recovered from it over the weekend, not over the following month.

She forgot—for hours at a time, and then for days—to think about her body.

She stopped bracing for consequences that never arrived.

It receded from the foreground of her attention and became the background of her life. Something she lived inside rather than something she managed.

The binder is in a closet somewhere.
She has not opened it in years.
That is what healing in order makes possible.
Let us begin.

CHAPTER ONE

The Right Treatment at the Wrong Time

"The question is never whether the
treatment is correct in theory.
The question is whether the body is ready to receive it.
And the answer to that question depends entirely
on where you are in the sequence."
—Marcus Ettinger, DC

A Note on Patient Stories: The patient stories in this book are composite clinical narratives drawn from recurring patterns observed across many patients over 37 years of practice. Names, identifying details, and specific circumstances have been blended and modified to protect privacy while preserving the physiologic patterns central to the Ettinger Foundation Protocol (EFP) framework. Any resemblance to a specific individual is coincidental. These narratives are true in the way that matters most: they reflect what actually happens to real people, again and again, in predictable and understandable ways.

Her name is Claire. She was forty-three years old when she first came to see me, and she arrived with a binder.

Not an unusual binder. Not a thin folder of insurance forms and a recent lab panel. A three-inch binder, organized by category: test results going back eleven years, printed summaries from twelve different practitioners, a hand-typed timeline of every treatment she had tried and when she had tried it, and a section at the back she called, with a kind of exhausted precision, "Things That Made Me Worse."

That last section was the longest one.

If you have been chronically ill long enough, you may already know exactly what that section contains.

The treatments listed there were not fringe remedies. They were not the types of treatments a reasonable person would consider pseudoscience. They were treatments that genuinely helped people and were backed up by research—an anti-anxiety medication combined with a two-week antibiotic course her gastroenterologist had recommended, a mitochondrial-boosting supplement stack from a respected functional medicine practice, and an intensive adrenal recovery program from a naturopathic physician who had spent two hours reviewing her case. Each practitioner had been thoughtful. Each recommendation had made clinical sense. And each one, in Claire's words, had "taken me down."

Before she described what "taken me down" meant clinically, she told me what it meant in her life.

She had been a project manager for a mid-sized architecture firm. Past tense. She had gone part-time three years earlier when the combination of fatigue and unpredictable digestive symptoms had made full-time work unsustainable. She had gone home-based two years after that. She had not been to the office—any office, for any reason—in fourteen months. Not because she could not do the work. Because she could not trust her body to cooperate for an unpredictable number of hours in an unfamiliar bathroom situation.

The unpredictability of chronic alternating constipation and diarrhea had been the organizing factor of her daily life for just over four years. She had not eaten at a restaurant she had not previously vetted in two years—vetted meaning she knew where the bathroom was, knew she could leave quickly, and knew the menu well enough to identify the few things that would not predictably trigger a response. She had stopped attending her daughter's school events in the third and fourth grades. Not all of them—she had made it to the important ones, the ones her daughter would remember. But she had missed enough that her daughter, now eleven, had learned not to assume her mother would be there, which was its own kind of loss that Claire named carefully and set aside.

"I want to tell you what I've given up trying to explain to people," she said. "Because I've stopped explaining. It's easier to just not go."

She had stopped explaining because the explanation was too long, too conditional, and too dependent on variables that changed from week to week. She had stopped making plans more than a day in advance because plans required a body she could predict, and her body had stopped being predictable years ago.

What had replaced planning was another form of cognitive work—the constant, invisible calculation that chronically ill people know intimately and that healthy people almost never have to perform. Before agreeing to anything, she ran a private assessment: How am I today? What did I eat yesterday? How far is the drive? Is there a bathroom I trust? What's the cost if I have to leave early? Can I recover before Tuesday? This calculation had become so automatic that she no longer experienced it as a decision. It was just the first thing her mind did when someone asked her to be somewhere.

Her social life had contracted to the people who would come to her, on her terms, in an environment she could control.

"What does my future look like if this doesn't change?" She said it flatly, like she had rehearsed it. "My daughter is eleven. She'll be in high school in three years. I want to go to her games. I want to take the trip we've been talking about since she was seven. I want to go back to work in an office doing work I'm good at. I want to make a plan and trust that I'll be able to keep it. Right now, none of that is possible. And I don't know how much more of my life I can give to something that nobody seems to be able to explain."

She looked at me across the desk and said something I have heard, in one form or another, hundreds of times: "I don't understand why things that are supposed to help me make me feel so much worse."

That question is one of the reasons I wrote this book.

Before I answer it—before I explain what was actually happening to Claire and what is most likely happening to you—I want to acknowledge something.

If you are reading this book, there is a reasonable chance that you have been unwell for quite a while. That the experience of being unwell has been, in its own way, as exhausting as the illness itself. Not just the fatigue or the pain or the digestive chaos or the sleep that does not restore you—but the experience of seeking help, being told you are fine, trying the next thing, getting worse or not responding, and slowly arriving at a quiet and terrible suspicion that your body has become something you can no longer predict or trust.

Your body is not behaving randomly. It only feels random from inside the confusion.

It follows patterns that make physiologic sense once the sequence is understood. What appears to be random, treatment-resistant, or inexplicable does have a governing logic. I have spent close to four decades learning to recognize it.

That logic has a name. I call it the regulatory hierarchy: the order in which the body must restore stability before deeper healing can occur. And once you understand it, everything that has happened to you—especially the things that made you worse—will start to make sense.

The Central Idea

Here is the idea at the heart of this book, stated as plainly as I know how to say it:

Your body heals in a fixed biological order. Each layer of recovery depends on the stability of the one beneath it. When you try to heal a later phase before an earlier one is stable, the treatment fails—or worse, it makes you worse. This is not a mystery. It is physiology.

The human body is not a collection of separate systems that can be tuned independently. It is a hierarchy of phases, each one dependent on the stability of the phase below it. At the base is the autonomic foundation—the part of the nervous system that continuously determines whether the body can regulate, recover, and adapt, or whether it must protect and conserve. Above that is immune regulation. Above that is the circadian system and the sleep-driven repair it enables. Above that is cellular energy production. And above that, finally, is structural repair—the rebuilding of strength, resilience, and physical capacity.

These phases do not operate on a timeline of your choosing. You cannot redirect the body's energy toward mitochondrial activation while your autonomic system is still in high-alert conservation mode. You cannot fully repair the gut lining while inflammatory signals are still degrading it. You cannot rebuild structural tissue while your circadian clock is too disrupted to generate the hormonal pulses that tissue repair depends on at night. The phase hierarchy reflects biological order rather than a clinician's preference. The sequence is not adjustable.

Most people discover this only after years of trying things that should have helped.

The right treatment, applied to the wrong phase, does not simply fail to work. In an unstable system with limited recovery capacity, it often makes things worse.

This is what happened to Claire. Every treatment she received was, in principle, appropriate. The antibiotic protocol addressed a medical diagnosis of IBS. The mitochondrial support was targeting genuine energy dysfunction. The adrenal recovery program was responding to a real hormonal pattern in her data. But each was aimed at a phase that her body had not yet reached in its own recovery sequence. And when you ask an already-overloaded system to process one more active input, the system does not have the recovery capacity to absorb it. It amplifies its threat response. You feel worse.

What Claire needed was treatment aimed at the foundation. Not the most sophisticated treatment. The earliest one. The one her body had sufficient recovery capacity to receive.

Why Correct Treatments Worsen Unstable Systems

This concept deserves a more direct explanation than most books in this category provide. Because "the right treatment at the wrong time can make you worse" sounds like clinical philosophy until you understand the mechanism. The mechanism is not philosophical. It is physiologic.

When the body is under sustained physiologic stress—managing a regulatory imbalance for months or years—it progressively shifts its resource allocation away from growth, repair, and performance toward protection and conservation. This is not dysfunction. This is adaptive intelligence.

In this state, the body's physiologic bandwidth—its available capacity for processing inputs, coordinating responses, and adapting to change—is already largely committed. The immune system is maintaining active surveillance. The autonomic system is holding a threat-ready posture. The mitochondria are operating in energy-conservation mode. The circadian system is generating a degraded but functional rhythm. Every available resource is allocated.

Now introduce a treatment. Any treatment—a probiotic, a mitochondrial cofactor, an antimicrobial protocol, or a hormone support formula. Each of these is physiologically active. Every physiologically active input sends signals throughout the body. In physiology, signaling is simply the way one part of the body communicates with another about what to do next. Those signals require a coordinated response—activate or suppress, repair or conserve, grow or defend. Each new treatment therefore represents an additional demand on a system that has no spare capacity to meet it. The additional input is not received as therapeutic support—it is experienced as increased demand on an already-constrained system. The autonomic system interprets increased demand as increased threat. Protective signaling intensifies. Symptoms worsen.

This is why so many chronically ill people eventually become afraid of treatment itself.

Their experience has taught them something accurate: treatments that help other people consistently make them feel worse. That experience is not psychological. It reflects the physiology of a system that is already operating at its limit. Once you understand the mechanism, the pattern becomes entirely predictable.

This distinction—between a treatment being correct in principle and a system being ready to receive it in practice—is the clinical insight at the center of this book. It explains why so many people accumulate a long history of treatments that were individually appropriate but collectively unsuccessful: they were introduced before the body had established the foundation required to benefit from them.

The Man Who Ran Every Morning

Not everyone who comes to see me has a binder. Some of them, at least from the outside, look like they are doing everything right.

David was fifty-one. He had been an athlete his entire adult life—not competitive, but consistent. He ran four or five mornings a week, ate carefully, slept what he thought was enough, and had the blood panel to prove that something was working. His inflammatory markers were fine. His thyroid was fine. His testosterone was in range. His doctor had told him on every visit that he was in excellent health for his age.

And yet for the previous two years, something had been wrong.

He could not describe it with clinical precision. It wasn't pain or dramatic fatigue. It was more like a ceiling he kept running into—a sense that his body was no longer responding the way it used to. He would finish a run feeling like he had done twice the distance. He would sleep eight hours and wake up tired. He would have a productive day and pay for it over the next two. He began structuring his weeks around the knowledge that certain kinds of effort would cost him the following day, which meant that his calendar had become a map of anticipated debt.

What the ceiling was costing him was harder to describe than the ceiling itself. Running for David was not simply exercise. It had been his primary tool for managing stress, processing difficulties, and maintaining his sense of himself as someone physically capable and in control of his own body. He had run through his father's illness. He had run through a professional setback that had cost him two years of work. He had run through the transition to an empty house when both his children left for college within the same year. Running had always been the thing that reliably returned him to himself—the practice that converted a hard day into a manageable one, that turned stress into something his body could metabolize and release.

And now the predictability was gone. The run that had always been the solution was becoming part of the problem. This left him without a way to get back to himself. Without a tool he knew how to use.

"I'm doing everything I've always done," he said. "Why is it suddenly not working?"

The labs showed nothing. His doctor suggested stress. His wife suggested he was getting older or working too hard. He came to me because neither explanation felt right—and because somewhere in those two years of accumulated confusion, he had begun to suspect that something real was happening to him that nobody had yet been able to name.

He was correct.

The answer was not that his habits had stopped working. It was that the regulatory foundation beneath those habits had shifted—quietly and gradually, over years—in a way that his labs could not detect and his doctor had no framework for. His autonomic system had been running a low-grade protective state for long enough that it had changed the conditions under which his mitochondria could operate adaptively. Not broken—recalibrated. Shifted from adaptive mode to conservation mode, because the signals they were receiving said that conservation was the appropriate response to the current physiologic environment.

In this context, his running was no longer functioning as the adaptive stimulus it had always been. It was now functioning as a demand that his system could not fully recover from. Each session was adding to a recovery debt that was never fully cleared. The debt was compounding. And eventually, the debt became the ceiling.

His body was no longer adapting. It was compensating.

The solution was not to stop running. It was to understand that his body had changed the conditions under which running could be adaptive—and to address those conditions before asking his body to perform.

Why Medicine Misses This

Claire had seen twelve practitioners. David's doctor had told him he was in excellent health. Both were receiving care from competent, well-trained clinicians who had access to sophisticated diagnostics and a genuine commitment to helping them. And yet the pattern—the sequence recovery depends on, the way upstream instability generates downstream symptoms, the way timing determines whether a treatment helps or harms—was invisible to all of them.

This is not a failure of intelligence or effort. It is a structural consequence of how modern medicine was built.

The great advances of twentieth-century medicine were built on reductionism: the disciplined isolation of specific mechanisms, the identification of specific pathogens, and the targeting of specific receptors. This approach produced extraordinary results for acute illness—bacterial infections, surgical emergencies, traumatic injuries. Discrete problems with identifiable causes and targetable solutions.

Reductionism works brilliantly when the problem is clearly defined and localized.

Chronic illness is most often neither localized nor clearly defined. It is a network problem—a disruption of regulatory coordination across multiple interdependent systems, expressed differently in different patients, resistant to single-target treatments because the target is not a specific pathogen or a specific deficiency. It is a sequence—an interconnected network of systems that have lost their coordinated function and must be restored in the order of their interdependence.

The problem is not which system appears to be affected. It is that the coordination between systems has broken down.

Medicine's organizational structure does not support this kind of thinking. Specialists are trained to see and treat the system that is their domain. The gastroenterologist sees the gut. The rheumatologist sees the immune system. The endocrinologist sees the hormones. The neurologist sees the nervous system. Each is seeing something real. Each is treating something real. And each stays in their lane.

What no single specialist is positioned to see is the upstream driver generating the findings across all of those domains simultaneously—because that upstream driver is not in any single system. It is in the regulatory relationship between systems.

Patients leave these appointments with more findings but less clarity. The body becomes more confusing, not less. People start collecting explanations instead of recovering.

This is not a failure of the practitioners. It is a failure of the framework they were trained inside.

Functional and integrative medicine improved on this by looking across systems—by asking what multiple findings might share as a common upstream cause. But even sophisticated functional approaches often identify what is dysregulated without fully accounting for when to address it. The adrenal finding is real. The mitochondrial finding is real. The gut finding is real. But treating them without first establishing the regulatory stability required to receive them is the same reductionist error, in a more sophisticated form.

The question has changed from "what system is affected?" to "what upstream mechanism is driving it?" But the equally important question—"what is the body ready to receive, and in what order?"—is still largely absent.

Diagnostic testing contributes to this gap. Regulatory instability often begins long before standard laboratory testing becomes abnormal.

A disruption of autonomic regulation means the body's automatic control systems no longer coordinate smoothly, making digestion, heart rate, blood pressure, temperature regulation, and stress responses less predictable. Chronic immune activation is the persistent activation of the body's protective alarm system, generating ongoing inflammatory signals that gradually interfere with recovery. A disruption of circadian amplitude means the body's daily rhythms lose their normal strength, making restorative sleep, hormonal timing, and repair less reliable. A disruption of mitochondrial efficiency means cells become less effective at converting nutrients into usable energy, leaving the body with less capacity for recovery, adaptation, and sustained function.

A standard lab panel can appear entirely normal while the systems responsible for regulation have already begun to lose their coordinated function.

The labs are not wrong.

They are not measuring the level at which the problem is occurring. They are looking for pathology in individual systems when the problem is in the regulatory coordination between them.

The test was normal. The patient was not.

The body's most important question in chronic illness is not "which system is damaged?" It is "where did regulatory stability break down first, and what must be restored before the next layer can recover?" That question requires a framework that medicine, as currently organized, is rarely positioned to ask.

What They Share

Claire and David are different people with different presentations and different histories. What they share—what I have seen across thousands of patient encounters—is a version of the same underlying problem.

Their bodies were responding appropriately to conditions that had made normal responses unsustainable. The autonomic nervous system was becoming less tolerant of demand and more protective—the expected response to sustained physiologic load. The immune system was maintaining heightened surveillance because the regulatory signals required to resolve the perceived threat had not been restored. The mitochondria were shifting toward energy conservation, preserving function while protecting the system from demands they no longer interpreted as safe to meet.

Claire and David were not responding abnormally. The conditions that generated those protective responses had been present for so long, and had been addressed so repeatedly at the level of the symptoms rather than the physiology that produced them, that the protective responses themselves had become the presenting symptoms. Treatment was aimed at those symptoms while the regulatory conditions generating them remained unchanged.

This is one of the central gaps in chronic illness care, and it is larger than any one practitioner or specialty. Modern medicine is extraordinarily good at identifying problems inside individual systems, but far less equipped to recognize what happens when instability begins in the relationship between those systems.

Most patients with chronic illness do not have a single isolated problem. They have a disruption in coordination across multiple layers of physiology. Sleep changes. Energy changes. Digestion changes. Stress tolerance changes. Recovery changes. The symptoms appear separate because they are expressed through different systems, but they are often being driven by the same upstream instability.

A bad night's sleep can affect digestion the next morning. Digestive disruption can increase physiologic stress. Stress can reduce recovery. Recovery debt accumulates until the body stops responding the way it once did. None of these changes is ever random. They are linked. And once enough layers are involved, the person no longer experiences a single problem. They experience a life that feels increasingly unpredictable.

This is why so many people with chronic illness eventually feel as though everything in their body is becoming connected to everything else. Because it is.

What often disappears first is resilience. Then recovery becomes less reliable. Then energy becomes inconsistent. Then sleep becomes lighter or less restorative. Then digestion becomes more reactive. Then the whole system becomes increasingly intolerant of stress, stimulation, unpredictability, or demand.

The symptoms can vary from person to person. The pattern underneath them often does not.

A practitioner who understands how to read that pattern can identify not only what has gone wrong, but what needs to be restored first. This book will show how to recognize where the sequence lost stability, what that disruption makes impossible further up the hierarchy, and what the system must regain before recovery can continue.

This pattern crosses all diagnostic categories because it is not a disease pattern. It is a physiologic pattern—the pattern of a recovery sequence that has been disrupted and then addressed out of order.

I see it in patients with autoimmune conditions and in patients with no diagnosis at all. I see it in patients who have been ill for decades and in patients who became ill just months ago after a viral infection they could not fully recover from. I see it in patients whose labs are dramatic and in patients whose labs are entirely normal.

The diagnosis changes.

The pattern does not.

What I Have Learned

Early in my career, I made the same mistakes that many practitioners make. I treated the loudest complaint. I chased the most elevated lab finding. I followed the research-backed protocols for the condition the patient appeared to have. And I watched with growing frustration as many patients who should have improved either stayed the same or even got worse—while others on the exact same protocol improved predictably.

The discrepancy bothered me enough that I started keeping detailed notes on it. Not the patients who improved—that was the expected outcome, and I documented them accordingly. The patients I tracked meticulously were the ones who worsened on treatments that should have helped. I wanted to understand the pattern of failure as precisely as I understood the pattern of success.

The turning point didn't come from a new study. It came from a patient I'll never forget. She was in her late thirties and had already seen multiple practitioners. She had tried every treatment her presentation seemed to call for. Instead of improving, her condition got worse—measurably and consistently—with each successive treatment.

I sat with her chart many times over the following days. The pattern I had been trying to explain away—patients worsening on "correct" treatments—wasn't an anomaly. It was the most consistent finding in the chart. And data that consistent is never incidental.

What I was seeing took me years to fully comprehend. But the beginning of that comprehension was simple: the responses were not random at all. They were predictable. The same treatments, applied to similar patients at similar points in their illness journey, consistently produced the same outcomes. There was a logic to it. It was a sequence. An order the body was insisting upon, regardless of the practitioner's plan.

What I eventually came to understand was that the body was following an order whether I recognized it or not. Recovery was unfolding from the foundation upward, according to biological dependency rather than clinical convenience. Whenever I introduced a treatment that belonged later in that sequence before the earlier layers had regained stability, the pattern was remarkably consistent. Patients stalled, relapsed, or deteriorated—not because the treatment was wrong, but because their physiology was not yet ready to receive it.

Over the years that followed, I developed the clinical framework on which this book is based. The central principle is not what to treat. It is when, and in what order.

That understanding can be stated in one sentence.

The sequence is the therapy. The timing is the treatment.

What This Book Is—and What It Is Not

If you have been ill for a long time, there is a good chance you have already accumulated lists of supplements, medications, diets, and treatment protocols that were supposed to help.

Some probably did.

Some may have helped for a while before the improvement faded.

Others may have made you feel noticeably worse.

That history is one of the reasons this book does not begin with another protocol.

A treatment has meaning only within the physiologic conditions in which it is introduced. The same intervention can be restorative for one person, ineffective for another, and overwhelming for someone whose recovery has not yet reached the point where that treatment can be successfully absorbed. The question is not whether a treatment is good. It is whether the body is ready to benefit from it.

That is why this book begins with understanding instead of prescriptions.

My goal is not to tell you what to take. It is to help you understand why treatments succeed, why they fail, and why the same intervention can produce remarkably different outcomes in different people.

Once that framework becomes clear, your own history begins to look different. Treatments that seemed random begin to reveal a pattern. Setbacks become information instead of mystery. And conversations with the practitioners helping you become more focused because you understand not only what is being recommended, but why it may—or may not—be the right next step.

Throughout this book, the word *healing* is used in a specific operational sense. It does not mean perfect health or the complete disappearance of every symptom. It means the measurable restoration of physiologic function: increasing predictability, improved recovery, greater resilience, restored tolerance, and a body that once again adapts more easily to the demands placed upon it.

That is what healing in order means.

Where We Are Going

In the chapters that follow, I will walk you through the phase hierarchy. It is a physiologic map of what your body is trying to do and why it sometimes cannot.

We will start at the foundation and work upward through each phase, in the order the body requires. At each phase, we will meet composite patients whose experiences make the physiology recognizable. We will look at what that phase requires from the one below it, what it makes possible for the one above it, and what the most common clinical mistakes look like when a phase is misaddressed or skipped.

Along the way, we will examine why the pattern of treatment failure in chronic illness is so consistent—and why understanding it as a sequencing problem rather than a treatment problem changes everything about what comes next.

This book was written for people living with chronic illness. But the framework it describes applies whenever recovery begins to lose its normal biological order. For some people, that unfolds gradually over months or years. For others, it begins much more abruptly following a viral illness or another major physiologic stress. The sequence of recovery is the same. What differs is the depth of the disruption and the patience the timeline requires.

Claire made a full recovery. It took nearly two years and demanded a level of patience she wasn't sure she possessed. But this was real recovery—not merely managed, compensated, or maintained through ongoing treatments. It was the kind of healing that eventually allowed her to stop thinking about her body and simply live inside it again.

She went back to the office. She took the trip with her daughter. She trusted her body enough to make plans again.

What recovery looked like, in practice, was not dramatic. It was the absence of the calculation. The unpredictable became predictable. She made a dinner reservation without first mapping the exit. She said yes to things without consulting an internal ledger of energy reserves. She had a difficult week and recovered from it over the weekend, not over the following month. She forgot—for hours at a time, and then for days—to think about her body. She stopped bracing for consequences that never arrived. It receded from the foreground of her attention and became the background of her life.

The binder is in a closet somewhere. She has not opened it in years.

That is what healing in order makes possible.

Let us begin.

CHAPTER TWO

The Body Is Not a List of Problems

"When we treat the symptom, we are answering a question the body has not actually asked. The body's question is always about order."
—Marcus Ettinger, DC

The way we approach the human body is built on hundreds of years of scientific discovery and has transformed the practice of medicine. Yet, in the care of chronic illness, it has also become the source of many failures I have spent my career trying to understand.

It goes like this: the body is a collection of systems. The digestive system. The immune system. The hormonal system. The nervous system. The cardiovascular system. Each system has its own specialists, diagnostic tests, and treatments. When a system malfunctions, you identify the problem. Medicine becomes the process of identifying isolated malfunctions and correcting them.

This model works extraordinarily well for a certain category of illness. If you break your leg, the orthopedist sets the bone and it heals. If you develop a bacterial infection, the antibiotic eliminates the bacteria and you recover. The problem is discrete. The solution is targeted. The body complies.

Chronic illness is not like this.

In chronic illness—the persistent, multi-system, treatment-resistant type that fills the waiting rooms of integrative medicine practices and the comment sections of patient support groups—the symptoms do not behave like discrete problems with discrete solutions. The gut is inflamed. The immune system is overactive. The joints ache. Sleep is disrupted. Energy is unreliable. The brain is foggy. The same treatment that calmed the gut last month is now making everything worse. When you address one problem, another one moves. When you suppress one symptom, two others intensify.

Patients who live with this experience often arrive at the same conclusion: that their body has lost its internal coordination. That there is no coherent explanation for what is happening to them.

They are right that the conventional medical model has no explanation. There is one. It just requires a different way of understanding what the body actually is.

Five Diagnoses. One Pattern

Her name is Elena. She was thirty-eight years old and had been a dedicated high school biology teacher for twelve years when she first came to see me. There was a weary awareness in her voice. She had spent her career explaining cellular biology to teenagers, and could not explain what was happening inside her own body.

She was not someone who described symptoms easily. What she described instead was a before and an after—and the gap between them.

Before: she had not taken a sick day in twelve years. She coached the Science Olympiad team, ran an after-school club, and drove forty-five minutes each way because she believed in the district where she taught. She ran three mornings a week. When a student was struggling, her colleagues knew they could count on her. She was the person who stayed late, volunteered first, and almost never had to wonder whether she would have enough energy for what the day asked of her.

After: she stepped down from coaching eight months ago because she could not predict, from one afternoon to the next, whether she would have the energy to stay past the final bell. She dropped the after-school club and was considering, with considerable grief, whether she could continue teaching at all.

"I keep waiting for it to plateau," she said. "For the decline to stop somewhere and hold. But it doesn't plateau. Every few months there's something else I can't do that I could do before."

What she was describing was the experience of living at sixty percent of her capacity, consistently, without any single moment catastrophic enough to explain why she had to give up so many of the things she once did.

Her digestion had become what she called "the unpredictable factor in every decision I make." She had developed chronic diarrhea that followed no pattern she could identify. When she went somewhere new, the first thing she did was locate the exits and the bathrooms. She had declined invitations to two conferences and turned down an offer to serve as the keynote speaker at a regional education summit—work she had been building toward for years—because she could not trust her body through an entire day away from a known environment.

"I haven't told my husband how much I've stopped doing," she said. "He knows some of it. He doesn't know all of it. I don't want him to see how much I've lost."

She paused.

"What does my future look like if this doesn't change? Do I become someone who used to do things? I am thirty-eight years old. I had assumed I had at least another thirty years of being the person I worked so hard to become. I don't want to spend them becoming less of myself."

Over the course of her illness she had accumulated five diagnoses: irritable bowel syndrome, generalized anxiety disorder, probable small intestinal bacterial overgrowth, subclinical hypothyroidism, and a finding on an autoimmune panel her rheumatologist described as "worth watching but not yet actionable." Each diagnosis was real. Each treatment was appropriate for what it addressed. And none of them, individually or in combination, produced any sustained improvement.

"Every specialist I see gives me a piece of the puzzle. But nobody has the box."

That sentence has stayed with me. It describes, with more precision than most clinical explanations, what the reductionist model of medicine often cannot provide: the picture that shows how the pieces fit together.

What Elena had was one upstream pattern of instability expressing itself across five layers of physiology at once. The five diagnoses described where that instability was being expressed. They did not describe the single pattern connecting them. And understanding that—the sequence her body was following—is what this chapter is about.

What the Body Actually Is

The human body is not a collection of independent systems. It is an ordered sequence of dependent layers, each one resting on the stability of the one below it.

Most people understand this intuitively about buildings. A building does not just need the right materials placed in the right rooms. It needs a foundation before walls, and walls before a roof. The sequence is a structural necessity. Load moves downward. What is below determines what is possible above.

The body works the same way—but with one important difference. Buildings are static. The body is dynamic. It continuously monitors its own state, makes decisions about resource allocation, and adjusts what it invests in based on what it perceives the situation to require. When conditions are stable, it invests in growth, repair, and performance. When conditions are unstable, it redirects those resources toward protection and conservation.

Buildings illustrate why sequence matters. A municipal power grid illustrates how the body manages that sequence in real time.

A functioning power grid matches supply to demand in real time. When demand increases, it routes more power. When a component fails, it reroutes around the failure. When supply is constrained, it prioritizes essential loads and sheds non-essential ones. It is a coordinated system that maintains balance across all of its components simultaneously.

Now imagine a power grid under sustained stress—a region that has been running at ninety percent of capacity for months. The transmission lines are still working. The generators are still running. The lights are still on. But there is no reserve. Every time an additional load comes online, the system cannot absorb it. Circuit breakers trip. Brownouts occur. Regions that seemed stable become unstable. And the problem is not in any single component. It is in the relationship between supply and demand across the entire system.

That is the body in chronic illness. Not a broken system. An overloaded one, rerouting constantly, conserving where it can, protecting what it must, with no reserve left for the growth and repair it was designed to sustain.

The treatments that should help often don't because they represent an additional load on a system with no spare capacity. The circuit breakers trip. You feel worse. The breaker isn't the problem. It is telling you the system has reached its limit.

This is the operating logic of human physiology. It is why treating one system in isolation so rarely produces lasting improvement in chronic illness.

The systems do more than coexist. They borrow from one another, compensate for one another, and suppress one another under strain. When the nervous system remains in a sustained protective state, it directly reshapes immune behavior—increasing inflammatory signaling, disrupting gut motility, and lowering the body's tolerance for new inputs. When immune activation remains elevated for long enough, it begins interfering with sleep architecture, energy regulation, and the hormonal signals that govern daily rhythm. And when energy conservation becomes the body's default posture, mood, cognition, digestion, and stress tolerance all adjust accordingly.

None of these changes occurs in isolation. Each is a downstream consequence of instability somewhere earlier in the sequence. Treating the downstream consequence may temporarily reduce the symptom, but it does not change the upstream conditions that continue generating it. As long as those conditions remain in place, the body continues producing the same protective responses. The symptom returns. Patients experience partial improvement, temporary relief, and eventually find themselves back where they started.

A Map of the Sequence

Before we go any further, let me show you the entire recovery sequence. Seeing the whole map first will make it easier to understand why each phase depends on the one beneath it. Throughout this book, "phase" refers to your position in the recovery sequence. "Layer" describes the dependency between phases—the way each phase is supported by the one below it. Each phase is introduced here with a brief description. Over the next six chapters, we'll examine each one in detail. Think of this as the map you'll return to throughout the rest of the book.

Phase	What it establishes
Phase 6: High-Level Coordination	Sustained, integrated function—output without drift (optional advanced clinical phase)
Phase 5: Structural Repair	Rebuilding strength, tissue, and physical resilience
Phase 4: Cellular Energy	Adaptive energy production—responsive to demand
Phase 3: Circadian Rhythm	Sleep-driven repair and daily timing of restoration
Phase 2: Immune Regulation	Gut stability, barrier integrity, and inflammatory resolution
Phase 1: Autonomic Foundation	Regulatory safety and flexibility

Nothing above Phase 1 holds without it.

Read the sequence from the bottom up, and you have the order in which recovery must occur. Read it from the top down, and you have the order in which function is lost when the system comes under sustained stress.

Top-down loss. Bottom-up recovery. That is the pattern. And it is consistent enough that, once you know it, you can recognize your own history of illness in it.

Here is something worth pausing on: the first symptom you noticed is almost certainly not the first thing that changed. By the time that change crosses the threshold of awareness and begins interrupting your daily life, the layer below has often been compromised for weeks or months.

The body compensates quietly and for longer than most people realize. It has redundant pathways, and it reroutes. It borrows from tomorrow's recovery budget to meet today's demands. The compensation works—until it doesn't. What patients experience as sudden illness is often accumulated instability that has finally exceeded the body's capacity to conceal it. What you experience as the beginning is usually already the middle. And that means the restoration sequence needs to start earlier than the symptom map suggests.

The Phases Are Not Permanent

There is one more thing the map cannot show, because a map has to hold still and a body does not.

Because the loss moved through these layers over time, your position in them is not fixed either. Throughout this book, a phase refers to the earliest layer whose instability is currently governing recovery. That is what it means to be "in" a phase: not that everything above it has failed and everything below it is behind you, but that this is the layer where the sequence is currently stalled—the place where recovery is waiting to resume.

You are not a Phase 2 patient. Your physiology is, for now, operating most like Phase 2. Those are different claims. The first is an identity, fixed and a little hopeless. The second is a description of where your body is standing today, and today is not permanent.

As the layers beneath become more stable, the body moves upward through the sequence. Recovery becomes more complete, energy more reliable, strength more sustainable. The phase you are operating from does not have to be where you remain.

Life can move the sequence in the other direction as well. A serious illness, a prolonged stretch of poor sleep, a bereavement, a surgery, a period of relentless stress—any of these can reduce the body's ability to hold the layers it had already established. Someone functioning well in a higher phase may begin, for a time, to express the characteristics of a lower one. This is not relapse in the sense of failure. It is biology responding to changed conditions, exactly as it did the first time.

The way back is the same sequence, beginning again from wherever the body now stands.

The sequence does not change. Your position within it can.

As you read the chapters that follow, you may recognize yourself in more than one phase. That is not a sign that the model is failing. It is a sign that recovery is a process rather than a snapshot—that you may have lived through more than one of these layers and may move through them again as your physiology and circumstances change. One phase may feel especially familiar because it reflects where your physiology is operating today. Others may belong to earlier seasons of your illness, or to times when recovery was already underway.

What Elena's Five Diagnoses Were Actually Saying

Return to Elena for a moment. Her five diagnoses map onto the sequence in a way that reveals precisely how one foundational pattern of instability can produce a clinical picture that looks, to every specialist involved, like five separate problems.

The irritable bowel syndrome—the chronic diarrhea, the food reactivity, the digestive unpredictability—reflected a Phase 2 pattern. These findings represented immune dysregulation, barrier compromise, and gut motility disruption driven by deeper autonomic instability. These were real findings. But not the origin.

The subclinical hypothyroidism reflected a Phase 3 pattern. Thyroid regulation is deeply influenced by circadian signaling. When the body's daily rhythm of hormonal output degrades, thyroid function becomes inconsistent. The lab finding was real. The interpretation—that it reflected a primary thyroid disorder requiring thyroid treatment—missed the underlying pattern driving the disruption.

The anxiety disorder reflected a compromised autonomic system. Not simply a primary psychiatric condition. The autonomic system was under sustained physiologic stress, and the cognitive and emotional symptoms were how that strain became consciously felt. Treating them as isolated psychiatric symptoms while leaving the physiologic foundation unaddressed produced only partial and temporary relief.

The autoimmune finding reflected a Phase 2 pattern, but the source lay in an earlier phase.

Throughout this book, I will call that upstream source a driver—the earlier phase responsible for the downstream problem.

Her immune system was responding to a nervous system that had not yet stopped signaling threat. Until that driver is addressed, the immune system can remain in chronic low-level activation, generating the inflammatory signaling that often precedes identifiable autoimmune disease.

And the fatigue and weight gain and lost resilience reflected Phases 3, 4, and 5 simultaneously—the circadian system unable to generate the restorative sleep the body needed, mitochondrial energy production in conservation mode, and the structural repair systems unable to maintain what the body was asking them to sustain.

Five diagnoses. Five phases of the sequence. One foundational pattern of instability: an autonomic foundation that had been in a sustained protective state long enough to compromise every layer above it.

None of Elena's practitioners were wrong about what they found. What they were missing was the order.

Elena's experience of this had a specific texture: the sense of a life that kept becoming smaller, managed down to a size the body could tolerate, without anyone ever explaining why the managing never ended.

Restricted Stability vs. True Stability

Not everyone who appears stable is actually stable. There is a distinction in clinical practice that I find myself making constantly, because its implications for treatment are significant. I call it the difference between restricted stability and true stability.

Restricted stability is what it sounds like. The patient is managing. Their symptoms are controlled. They may have gone months without a significant flare. From the outside, they seem to have found their footing.

But their stability is not internal—it is environmental. It depends entirely on a set of carefully maintained conditions: a restricted diet, a rigid schedule, the avoidance of specific triggers, the absence of anything unpredictable. Remove one variable and the system destabilizes quickly and significantly.

These patients have not recovered. They have contracted.

Think of what that contraction actually looks like in a life. First, the travel radius shrinks—they stop taking trips that require unfamiliar bathrooms, unpredictable food, or uncertain schedules. Then the social radius shrinks—they stop accepting invitations that cannot be controlled, stop going to events where leaving early would be noticed, stop making the spontaneous decisions that healthy people make without thinking. Then the dietary radius shrinks—fewer foods, fewer restaurants, fewer evenings out. Then the professional radius—fewer commitments, smaller roles, shorter days. Then the emotional radius—fewer risks, fewer new relationships, less willingness to put themselves in situations where the body might fail them publicly.

Not collapse. Contraction. Slow and systematic, barely perceptible from the outside. The person is still upright. Still functional. Still managing. But the life they are living has become a much smaller version of the life they once had, and the distance between the two grows a little each year.

Many patients believe they are getting better because they are flaring less. But they are flaring less because they are encountering fewer variables—not because their system has become more stable. Symptom reduction from restriction is not the same as symptom reduction from healing. They feel identical from the inside. They are physiologically opposite.

What makes restricted stability so difficult to recognize—in yourself or in someone you care about—is that it feels like wisdom. The restrictions feel earned. The routines feel protective. The avoidance feels prudent. After years of unpredictable responses to ordinary life, the discovery that careful control produces fewer symptoms can feel like a breakthrough. And in the short term, it is. The system is less stressed. The symptoms are quieter.

But the psychology of restriction becomes its own problem over time. The patient grows afraid of variability itself. Each successful avoidance reinforces the belief that the trigger—the food, the supplement, the place, the activity, the social engagement—was the danger, rather than the system's inability to absorb it. They begin organizing life around preservation rather than participation. And eventually, they mistake environmental control for physiologic recovery, because from the inside they feel about the same. The difference is visible only when the control is removed—which they are now afraid to do.

The patient who has learned to live within restricted stability is often the most difficult to treat—not because their case is the most complex, but because the adaptation itself has become invisible to them. They describe themselves as stable. They are. They are just stable within a radius so narrow that ordinary life sits outside it.

Clinicians make the same mistake. When a patient stops flaring, we tend to interpret that as improvement. But if the flare reduction coincides with a reduction in exposure to triggers, the system has not become more resilient. It has been shielded. Remove the shield and the system will respond exactly as it did before.

Families make the same mistake. They see the person managing and conclude the problem has passed. And when the person declines or disappears from the plan at the last minute, there is a small bewilderment—"I thought you were doing better"—that lands in the patient as one more piece of evidence that their experience is invisible.

True stability is something entirely different. It is not the absence of triggers. It is the presence of resilience—the capacity to encounter variation, to absorb the unexpected, and to return to baseline without cascading. A different meal this week. A disrupted sleep schedule. A stressful conversation. A day that runs longer than planned. True stability means these things happen and the system accommodates them.

The question that determines whether a patient is ready to advance in the recovery sequence is not "are they better?" It is "can their system absorb variation without losing its footing?" A patient who is only better when everything is controlled has not yet reached the stability required by the next phase. Building on restricted stability is like building on sand. It holds, until it doesn't.

Compensation Is Not the Same as Recovery

Restricted stability is what the system can tolerate. There is another pattern that describes the cost of staying within that range. I call it compensation, and it is where most of the daily work of living with chronic illness actually happens.

Compensation is the collection of strategies—some conscious, most not—that allow a compromised system to continue functioning at an acceptable level. Unlike restricted stability, which is about the narrowness of the system's tolerable radius, compensation is about the cost of staying inside it.

The extra cup of coffee that makes the morning cognitively possible. The rigid bedtime that prevents the sleep disruption that would take two days to recover from. The careful meal planning that heads off the digestive consequences. The deliberate rationing of social energy to protect the commitments that matter most. The pre-emptive rest days built into every schedule, because not having them costs more than the days themselves.

Each of these, individually, is reasonable. But taken together, they consume a significant portion of the person's available physiologic and cognitive bandwidth.

The person is not living their life. They are administering it.

And here is what makes compensation dangerous: it works. For a while, often for years, the compensatory strategies hold the system functional. The person can participate. They can perform. They can pass. And because the compensation works, neither the patient nor the practitioner looks closely at the cost.

The cost is this: every unit of physiologic capacity spent maintaining the compensatory structure is a unit that is no longer available for repair and rebuilding. The person is running a deficit—spending more on maintenance than the system is generating—and the deficit accumulates, slowly and invisibly, until the compensatory strategies begin to fail.

This is what borrowed capacity means. The body can temporarily maintain output by drawing on reserves that are meant for recovery. It can borrow from tonight's repair budget to get through this afternoon. It can borrow from next week's immune regulation to manage this week's stress. Each individual withdrawal is small. But the debt accumulates invisibly, in the way that only biological debts can—silently, without a statement arriving in the mail, until the day the account is empty and the body has nothing left to draw on. That is the moment patients typically appear in a clinical setting. Not at the beginning of the compensatory phase, when the strategies are working. At the end of it, when they are not.

The longer the compensatory structure is in place, the more it reshapes the person's relationship with themselves. They stop trusting spontaneity—the impulse to say yes to something unplanned becomes a source of anxiety rather than pleasure. They stop expecting their body to cooperate without management. They stop making the kind of plans that assume physical reliability and start making only the plans that have an exit. Over time they begin to see themselves differently—as someone whose primary job is to manage their own limitations rather than to participate in their own life. The illness does not have to be severe for this to happen. It just has to be long enough.

The clinical implication is straightforward but important: recovery cannot begin until compensation is recognized for what it is. Not coping. Not progress. Not stability. A temporary and resource-intensive bridge that the system is crossing at a cost that is not visible on the surface.

When Recovery Stalls

Patients plateau. They improve for a period—sometimes significantly—and then stop improving. The gains hold, but no further progress occurs. A new treatment is attempted and produces no effect, or produces a worsening that seems to erase the gains that had been made.

I know what patients think during a plateau. I have heard it hundreds of times, in dozens of variations. "Nothing is working." "I thought I was getting better." "The protocol stopped working." "Maybe this is as good as it gets."

None of these interpretations is correct. And in most cases, the plateau has a specific cause that is physiologic and understandable.

When a patient stalls between phases, the most common reason is that the phase below has not fully stabilized—not in its symptoms, but in its signaling. The autonomic system may appear improved. The lab markers may look better. The patient may be reporting that they feel more functional. But the underlying signal—the consistency and timing of what the layer below is sending up—is not yet reliable enough for the layer above it to build on.

Think of a radio station broadcasting intermittently. Sometimes the signal is clear. Sometimes it drops. The receiver is fine. The signal is not. And you cannot build stable reception on an intermittent signal, no matter how good the receiver is.

When the foundation broadcasts intermittently, the phases above it can improve during the periods when the signal is strong. But when the signal weakens, they drop with it. This is partial stability.

The improvement is real, but unstable. And from the inside, unstable improvement is almost impossible to distinguish from no improvement at all. The patient who has been improving for six weeks and then suddenly stops does not experience that pause as the body stabilizing the gains it has already made. They experience it as failure. The forward motion has stopped. The effort continues. This is the moment when many patients abandon the process entirely—not because the process has stopped working, but because the part of recovery that is working is now happening below the threshold of conscious experience.

In reality, the system is often consolidating its new level of stability—making it reliable enough that the body can safely build the next layer on top of it.

That consolidation often becomes visible only later, in retrospect, when the next layer begins to respond. Getting through the plateau requires understanding that the absence of visible progress is not the same as the absence of progress.

The clinical response to a plateau is always the same: return to the foundation and confirm that stability is truly established there. What is already there needs more time to stabilize before the layer above it can support what comes next.

Incomplete stability is not a treatment failure. It is a timing issue. And timing, as this entire book is about, is everything.

The Search for the One Thing

There is a pattern of thinking that often emerges during chronic illness, and it can become almost as burdensome as the illness itself.

When the body loses its internal coordination—when multiple systems begin expressing instability simultaneously—the mind responds with a search. Not for a framework. For a cause. One missing piece. The one thing that, if found and corrected, would finally make everything make sense.

The search takes many forms. The missing hormone. The hidden pathogen. The food sensitivity that nobody has identified yet. The genetic variant. The supplement that everyone else is responding to. The practitioner who will finally have the answer. Each new theory produces a brief surge of hope, then a treatment, then a result that is partial at best. Then the search resumes, a little more depleted than before.

This behavior is not irrational. It is the mind doing exactly what minds do: trying to force a systems problem into a single-cause model, because single-cause models are the only kind that offer the possibility of a single solution. The body is behaving like a network. The mind is searching for a single broken part. The tension between those two realities is exhausting.

Understanding the sequence does not eliminate the desire for one answer. But it reframes what the one thing actually is. The one thing is not a missing supplement or a hidden pathogen. The one thing is the phase of the sequence where stability was first lost. Find that, address that, and the downstream consequences begin to resolve as the system restores itself from the foundation upward.

Why the Order Matters So Much

The sequence is not just a description of how the body is organized. It is a description of what the body needs before it can accept help.

And "what it needs before it can accept help" is a concept that is almost entirely absent from the standard clinical conversation.

When you go to a practitioner with a problem, the implicit contract is: here is the problem, here is the treatment, the treatment addresses the problem, the problem resolves. This works when the problem is acute and the system is stable. The antibiotic works because your immune system is functional and the treatment tips the balance.

But when the system is not stable—when the foundation has been compromised by chronic stress, illness, or accumulated physiologic burden—the contract breaks down. The treatment is applied, but the conditions the treatment requires in order to work have not been established. And the system, which is already managing more than it can comfortably handle, experiences the additional treatment as demand rather than support.

The body is not broken when this happens. It is communicating.

And what it is communicating is not "this treatment is wrong." It is "I am not ready for this treatment yet." Learning to interpret that communication correctly—rather than treating it as failure or idiosyncrasy—is the foundational skill of healing in order.

Foundation Work You Can Do Now

Every chapter in this book ends with something concrete—a foundational practice, grounded in the same physiology we have been discussing, that you can begin without a prescription, without a practitioner, and without waiting until the rest of the picture is clear.

In this chapter, the practice is the simplest and most foundational one in the entire book. It is also the one that is most consistently skipped, underestimated, or deprioritized in favor of something that feels more active and more therapeutic.

The practice is this: pick one time to wake up each morning, and hold it.

Not approximately. Not when you can. Every day, including weekends, including days when sleep was poor, including days when you have nowhere to be until noon. The same time, within fifteen minutes, every day.

This sounds too simple to matter. It is not. Here is why.

Your circadian system is an entrainment system. It does not generate its rhythm in isolation. It generates it in response to timing cues from the environment, and the most powerful of those cues is light entering your eyes in the morning. The moment you wake and expose yourself to light—even the pale gray light of a cloudy day, ideally from outside or through an open window—you send a signal to the master clock in your brain that begins the twenty-four-hour cascade of hormonal and physiologic events that constitutes a day.

When that signal arrives at a consistent time each day, the cascade becomes predictable. The cortisol rise that energizes you in the morning strengthens. The melatonin that prepares you for sleep arrives at the right time in the evening. The immune system modulates on schedule. The gut moves at the right time. Everything the body does on a daily schedule runs more smoothly when the clock that governs it is consistently anchored.

When the wake time drifts—when you sleep in on weekends, stay up late, take irregular naps—the clock loses its anchor. The cascade becomes unpredictable. The body loses its rhythm. And everything in the sequence above the circadian layer runs less efficiently as a result.

What consistent wake time is doing, at a deeper level, is teaching the body predictability again. A body that has been operating in protective and compensatory mode has often lost the experience of being able to anticipate what is coming next. Consistent timing restores that anticipation—one morning at a time, one reliable signal at a time.

Consistency matters more than perfection. Missing one morning does not erase the progress of two weeks. A weekend of imperfect timing does not reset the clock to zero. The body responds to rhythm more than to intensity. A pattern held eighty percent of the time produces meaningful entrainment. What undermines the clock is not an occasional disruption—it is the absence of any consistent anchor at all. So hold the time when you can, return to it when you drift, and do not treat an imperfect week as a reason to abandon the practice. The clock responds to the overall signal, not to individual days.

You do not need to do anything else this week. Wake at the same time and expose your eyes to bright light within the first thirty minutes—outside if you can, through an open window if you can't, and bright artificial light if you wake before the sun. Spend some time outside whenever your day allows it. The body needs brightness, consistency, and timing. Then let light do what it has been doing for every living organism on this planet for four billion years.

Elena recovered. Not quickly, and not in a straight line. There were periods of real progress followed by plateaus that required returning to the foundation and consolidating before advancing. There were moments when the partial stabilization we discussed earlier made it feel like nothing was working.

But the direction held. And the day she walked in with the unmistakable ease of someone who had stopped managing every variable and started simply living, I thought of that first appointment. The careful past tense. The life she was becoming that she did not want to be.

She had coached the Science Olympiad team again that year. They had come in third at regionals. She had driven the forty-five minutes without once calculating whether she would be able to stay.

In the next chapter, we are going to look at the timing principle up close—the specific mechanism by which the right treatment, applied to the wrong phase, produces harm rather than healing. We will meet a patient whose experience of this is so precise and so recognizable that you may immediately think of someone you know.

But first: the wake time. Write it down. Hold it.

The sequence begins here.

CHAPTER THREE

Why the Right Treatment Made You Worse

"The sequence is the therapy.
The timing is the treatment.
The analysis is the intervention.
When and how determine outcome
more than what."
—Marcus Ettinger, DC

I want to tell you about a specific kind of appointment I've had many times throughout my career.

The patient arrives looking both hopeful and braced for disappointment—the particular expression of someone who has been here before, who has sat in this kind of chair in this kind of office and been given this kind of hopeful attention, and who has learned, through experience, to protect themselves from the hope while still showing up for the appointment.

They describe their history. The illness that started it—sometimes sudden, sometimes gradual. The practitioners they have seen. The treatments they have tried. And then, always, the part that is hardest to explain: the treatments that should have worked and didn't. Or worse—the treatments that should have worked and made everything worse.

I ask them to tell me about one of those. Just one, in detail.

What happened. What they had been told to expect. What actually happened instead. How long it lasted. Whether they went back to the practitioner who prescribed it, and if so, what that person said.

The answers to that last question are among the most consistent things in my practice. Because what practitioners almost universally say, when a patient reports that a treatment made them worse, is one of three things: that the patient must have had an underlying sensitivity to that specific compound; that they are experiencing a detoxification reaction and should push through; or, delivered with the particular combination of sympathy and uncertainty that characterizes a practitioner who does not have a better explanation: sometimes these things just happen.

None of these explanations is usually the full explanation. And the absence of a correct explanation leaves the patient in a position that is, in some ways, worse than the original symptom: not only are they unwell, they now have evidence from their own body that their body cannot be helped. That it responds to assistance with worsening. That there is something uniquely, inexplicably wrong with them.

There is not. And I am going to explain, in this chapter, exactly what is happening—because once you understand it, you will never again mistake your body's response to a treatment as evidence that your body cannot be treated.

James

His name is James. He was forty-six years old, a software engineer who had spent his career building systems that behaved predictably when correctly designed. His professional life was organized around a simple and deeply held principle: find the flaw in the logic, correct it, and the system performs as designed.

He brought that same methodology to his health—and it had served him well for most of his adult life. When something went wrong with his body, he researched it, found the most credible available explanation, identified the most evidence-supported treatment, and applied it carefully. This approach had worked for him repeatedly. It was how problems got solved.

The fatigue that began limiting his function three years before he came to see me did not respond to this approach. What troubled him almost as much as the illness itself was discovering that the way he had always solved problems no longer worked.

"I don't know how to be someone who can't figure something out," he said. "That's not a statement of arrogance. It's a statement of—I don't have another gear. Systematic problem-solving is what I do. And now it's not working."

He had not told anyone at work that he was struggling. Not his manager. Not his team. Not the colleagues he had worked alongside for a decade. He had learned to manage his presentation carefully—to schedule his most demanding cognitive work for the windows of his day when he was least impaired, to defer the rest, to appear, from the outside, like someone who was performing normally. The gap between how he appeared and how he felt had been widening for two and a half years. He described it as "performing a version of myself that I'm not sure I can sustain."

He had not told his wife the full picture either. She knew he was tired. She had watched him quietly stop doing the household projects he had always done on weekends, the cooking he had done on Sundays, the long Saturday morning runs that had been the organizing ritual of his week for fifteen years. She noticed the changes. She did not know how carefully he was calculating them. Each thing he stopped doing was something he had concluded he could no longer afford.

She also did not know that he had turned down a promotion six months earlier—not because he didn't want it, but because he did not trust himself to sustain the additional demands. He kept telling himself it was temporary. He told her it was about timing. The real reason was that he was rationing what he had left, and there was not enough to spare.

"I wasn't ready to give up," he said. "I just couldn't see another way through it." The promotion had become the first major thing he believed he could no longer afford. "I keep narrowing what I commit to. I keep finding the minimum viable version of each thing and doing that instead of the real thing. Eventually the minimum viable version of my life is just—existing. Functioning. Not living."

When he finally found a functional medicine practice that took his presentation seriously, he experienced what he described as the first genuine hope he had felt in two years. The testing was comprehensive. The analysis was sophisticated. The diagnosis—mitochondrial dysfunction with secondary adrenal insufficiency and significant gut dysbiosis—made sense of his symptoms in a way nothing had before. And the protocol that followed was exactly what a person with his findings should have received.

He took everything exactly as directed. He was, as he put it, "a model patient." Within ten days, he was the sickest he had ever been in his life.

What Was Actually Happening

Not the normal fatigue of his baseline illness. Something qualitatively different—a full-system worsening that he described as feeling like every system in his body had been turned up to a volume he could not tolerate. He could not sleep. His digestion, which had never been a major issue before, became chaotic. The brain fog that had been manageable became disabling. He developed what he described as a persistent sense of internal vibration—a feeling of physiologic agitation that he had never experienced before and could not explain.

He went back to his practitioner. He was told he was experiencing a die-off reaction—a Herxheimer response—and that pushing through was part of the process. He tried. After two more weeks of worsening, he stopped the entire protocol and spent the following six weeks recovering to his original, already-compromised baseline.

"I lost two months," he told me. "And I'm worse than I was before I started. Which means the thing I did to try to get better made me worse. Which means I can't trust my own judgment about what to try next. Which means I have no path forward that I can see."

What had happened to James was not a Herxheimer reaction. It was something more fundamental—and understanding it required looking not at what the protocol contained, but at what James's system was capable of receiving when the protocol began.

By the time James started his mitochondrial protocol, his nervous system had been in a sustained state of low-grade threat response for at least three years. His immune system was chronically activated, generating a background level of inflammatory signaling that was exhausting his physiologic reserves. His sleep had lost the deep restorative architecture that his cells depended on for repair. And his mitochondria, operating in a body under chronic inflammatory load and sleep deprivation, had shifted toward conservation mode—not because they were broken, but because the signals they were receiving said that conservation was appropriate.

This is the key point that James's original assessment missed: the mitochondrial dysfunction was real, but it was not primary. It was a downstream consequence of a system that had been operating in protective mode for years. The protocol targeted the mitochondria. It could not resolve the chronic threat physiology that had pushed them into conservation in the first place. As we discussed in Chapter 2, treating a downstream consequence while the upstream driver continues to generate it is precisely the pattern that produces the results James experienced.

The mitochondrial support protocol did exactly what it was designed to do: it increased mitochondrial signaling and metabolic output. In a regulated system with sufficient upstream stability, this is helpful. In James's system—whose nervous system was signaling danger and whose immune system was already managing a significant inflammatory load—higher mitochondrial output meant higher metabolic demand in a system already at its ceiling. The result was not improvement. It was amplification.

The antimicrobial protocol compounded this. Killing gut bacteria, even problematic ones, produces a rapid release of inflammatory bacterial cell wall components that the immune system must process. In a regulated immune system, this is manageable. In James's immune system, which was already activated and already resource-constrained, it was an additional demand that the system could not absorb without worsening.

But there was also a third mechanism operating in James that explained the specific and severe deterioration of his sleep—something that neither James nor his practitioners had connected to the gut protocol.

How Inflammation Blocks Sleep: The Tryptophan Diversion

When the immune system is chronically activated, generating a sustained background of inflammatory signaling, it does something to the body's chemistry that most practitioners never think to look for, but that has profound consequences for sleep, mood, and cognitive function.

Tryptophan is an amino acid obtained from food such as turkey, chicken, and eggs that the body uses to produce serotonin, and from serotonin, melatonin—the primary hormone that signals the body to begin the transition to sleep. Under normal conditions, dietary tryptophan moves through this pathway reliably, and the body generates the melatonin it needs at the right time each evening.

Chronic inflammation changes the way the body uses tryptophan. One way it does this is by activating an enzyme called indoleamine 2,3-dioxygenase (IDO), which diverts tryptophan away from the serotonin-melatonin pathway. Instead of supporting serotonin and melatonin production, tryptophan is redirected into an alternative pathway that produces compounds that increase arousal and make it harder for the brain to settle into the quiet state that sleep requires. This pathway is called the kynurenine pathway.

The consequence follows a recognizable pattern. A patient with chronic immune activation has chronic tryptophan diversion. Their melatonin signal is chronically reduced—not because their pineal gland is failing, but because the raw material it requires is being intercepted upstream. And the metabolites produced in its place actively oppose the neurologic conditions that sleep depends on.

This is not a sleep disorder in the conventional sense. It is an immune-driven suppression of the body's primary sleep-initiating chemistry.

And it explains why James's sleep became dramatically worse when his antimicrobial protocol increased his immune activation: more inflammation meant more IDO activity, which meant more tryptophan diversion, which meant less melatonin substrate, which meant that his already-impaired sleep architecture collapsed further.

This is why treating the immune system before the nervous system's foundation is stable, and treating sleep before the immune system is stable, consistently produces incomplete results. The layers are not independent. The biology flows in one direction. What happens earlier in the sequence determines what becomes possible later.

James's sleep was not a separate problem from his gut dysbiosis. It was a downstream consequence of the ongoing inflammation that the dysbiosis was driving. But the gut was not the highest layer in the sequence. Above it sat the nervous system conditions that were maintaining the immune activation and limiting recovery. Those conditions had not been addressed. The antimicrobial protocol targeted the place where the problem was visible, not the place where the sequence began. The result was exactly what the sequence predicts: increased physiologic demand, worsening sleep, and no meaningful improvement.

The treatments were right. The sequence was wrong. And in James's system, as in every system under chronic physiologic load, the sequence determined the outcome.

When Pushing Through Helps and When It Harms

Before we go further, one thing deserves direct attention: the instruction to push through.

Most patients with chronic illness have, at some point, been told that worsening symptoms during treatment are a sign the treatment is working.

That the body is detoxifying. That healing is uncomfortable and discomfort means progress. "Just push through it."

This is sometimes true. A new exercise program produces muscle soreness. A dietary change produces a temporary digestive adjustment. A shift in sleep schedule produces a few disrupted nights before the clock resets. These are examples of adaptive discomfort—the body responding to a new input and adjusting toward a new set point. The discomfort is real, but it is time-limited, proportional to the change being introduced, and followed by genuine improvement rather than baseline deterioration.

That was not what James experienced. It was systemic destabilization—a qualitatively different response in which multiple systems deteriorated simultaneously, the worsening extended well beyond the treatment period, and recovery returned him not to a new baseline but to his old one, six weeks later.

The distinction matters clinically. Adaptive discomfort passes within days and leaves the system better than it found it. Systemic destabilization spreads across systems, extends across weeks, and leaves the system depleted. From the inside, the difference is rarely subtle. Adaptive discomfort feels like work. Destabilization feels like losing ground.

Not every worsening means stop. But a worsening that crosses multiple systems simultaneously, that intensifies over days rather than resolving, that leaves you functioning below your prior baseline weeks after the treatment has stopped—that is the body communicating that the input exceeded its current capacity. The signal is not "push harder." It is "the foundation is not ready for this yet."

The Three Responses

When a treatment is applied to a system that is not ready to receive it, there are three possible outcomes. Understanding which one you have experienced—and why—is the first step toward understanding your own history of illness.

The first is no response. The treatment does nothing. The patient takes it, waits, and finds that nothing changes—for better or worse. This outcome gets dismissed as "it didn't work for me." But no response is not the same as an ineffective treatment.

Most patients interpret no response as evidence about the treatment: this approach doesn't work for my body. Most practitioners interpret it the same way and move on to the next treatment. What no response more often indicates is something about the sequence: the treatment was aimed at a real consequence while the conditions generating it remained unchanged. The floor has not been prepared. Whatever is placed on it will not stay. Addressing the gut, the hormones, or the mitochondria while the layer above them remains unstable produces exactly this result. Not worsening. Not improvement. The intervention arrives, the system cannot build on it, and nothing changes. The treatment was not wrong. It was aimed at the consequence rather than the conditions that generated it.

The second response is temporary improvement followed by return to baseline—or, in some cases, below it. The treatment works. Sometimes dramatically. The patient feels better in a way they haven't felt in months. They allow themselves, carefully, to hope.

And then it fades.

This is the response that insidiously erodes hope because it contains hope and then withdraws it. The patient has now experienced two things they cannot reconcile: their body can improve, but the improvement will not hold. The cycle often repeats. Improvement, collapse. Improvement, collapse. Each cycle extracts something that pure no-response does not: the patient begins to fear improvement, because they have learned that improvement is temporary and the return to baseline is coming.

What is actually happening in this response follows a consistent physiologic pattern. When a treatment addresses a real consequence, the system can temporarily improve. But the conditions sustaining the improvement have not changed. The visible finding returns. Imagine clearing a flooded room while the pipe feeding it remains broken. The floor dries. Then it floods again.

The third is worsening—the response James experienced and the response that carries the most lasting damage to a patient's relationship with treatment and with their own body. Temporary improvement teaches the patient that feeling better may not last. Significant worsening teaches them something deeper: that allowing themselves to hope may no longer feel safe.

What Worsening Does to a Person

James's statement—"I can't trust my own judgment about what to try next"—is the most important thing he said. More important, clinically, than any of the symptoms he described. Because it named the consequence that outlasts the worsening itself.

When a treatment makes you significantly worse, the immediate physiologic consequence is one thing. The psychological consequence is something else, and it lasts longer.

The patient who has experienced major worsening on a treatment stops approaching treatment hopefully. They begin approaching it defensively. Every new protocol, every new recommendation, every new suggestion from a practitioner or a friend or a book is evaluated first through the lens of the last time they tried something and it went wrong. The question is no longer "could this help me?" It is "how dangerous is this to try?"

Hypervigilance follows. The patient begins monitoring symptoms with an intensity that was not there before—not the ordinary monitoring of someone tracking their health, but the constant, exhausting scanning of someone who has learned that their body can turn on them without warning. Every sensation becomes a potential signal of impending destabilization. A slightly elevated heart rate. A new digestive symptom. A night of poor sleep. Each one that would have been unremarkable before the worsening now carries the question: is this the beginning?

The experimentation narrows. Where the patient might once have been willing to try a new approach with reasonable openness, they now require more certainty before attempting anything. The threshold for trying something new rises. They are aware they need help, unable to risk the help, caught between the certainty of continued illness and the fear of deliberate worsening.

And underneath all of this, for many patients, is something harder to name: the loss of trust in hope itself. Prior improvements that collapsed have taught them that feeling better is not safe—that it will be taken away. Patients begin to hold good days at a distance, not allowing themselves to feel the improvement fully because they have learned that full investment in improvement makes the collapse more devastating.

Hope has become dangerous.

And a patient who has stopped being able to hope is a patient whose recovery has been made more difficult by the very process of trying to recover.

This is the true wound underneath this chapter. Not the fatigue, not the insomnia, not the dysbiosis. It is this: the body can no longer be trusted to respond safely to help. And that loss of trust is not a personality trait or a failure of attitude. It is a learned response to a specific pattern of physiologic experience that nobody ever explained.

James carried all of this. The defensive approach to treatment, the hypervigilance, the narrowed experimentation, the careful management of hope. He had not named any of it when he came to see me—he described it through its behavioral consequences rather than its emotional ones. But it was present in every sentence about his history. And before anything else could change, it needed to be named.

Understanding why the worsening happened—not as a mystery or a personal failure but as a precise physiologic consequence of a correct treatment applied to an unready system—was the first therapeutic act. Not a treatment. An explanation. The explanation that allowed him to stop interpreting his history as evidence about his body's capacity and start interpreting it as information about sequence.

Why This Is Not Your Fault

I want to be explicit about something that rarely gets said clearly enough to those being treated for a chronic illness.

The experience of getting worse on treatments that should have helped is one of the most isolating experiences in chronic illness. It carries a weight of implied personal failure—as if the body's inability to respond to treatment reflects some deficiency of character, some failure of commitment, some unwillingness to get well. Practitioners contribute to this, often unintentionally, when they frame treatment failure as something to push through or a sensitivity to work around—frameworks that locate the problem in the patient's body as though it were a quirk rather than a meaningful physiologic signal.

For James, the failure was particularly destabilizing for reasons we named earlier in this chapter. But beneath the identity wound was something more fundamental and more universal: a body that had been trying, in the only language available to it, to communicate that it needed something different. That communication was misread as failure. It was not.

When your body responds to a treatment with worsening, it is demonstrating that its regulatory capacity is fully committed to maintaining its current level of function. There is no reserve available for processing additional inputs. This is not a character flaw. It is a direct consequence of what prolonged physiologic stress does to the body's ability to regulate over time. The body has been protecting itself. That protection has been so sustained and so total that it has consumed the spare capacity that recovery requires.

What it requires is not a stronger treatment. It requires an earlier one. One aimed at the foundation. One that the system is actually capable of receiving—because it is designed, specifically, to reduce the physiologic burden rather than add to it.

Only then can the body begin to recover in the order it was designed.

Borrowed Capacity

In the previous chapter, we introduced the concept of borrowed capacity—the body's ability to temporarily maintain function by drawing on reserves that are meant for recovery rather than performance. James's history is the clearest illustration of what borrowed capacity looks like in practice, and what happens when it runs out.

For three years before his mitochondrial protocol, James had been functioning—not at the level he was accustomed to or expected of himself. He was just getting by. He was getting to work. He was managing his responsibilities. He was holding the shape of his life in place, even as the things that made his life his—the weekend projects, the Sunday cooking, the Saturday runs—simply fell away.

He was doing this by borrowing. Every day that exceeded his genuine recovery capacity was a day that drew on the reserve he had been building across healthier years. The reserve was not visible. It produced no readout. But it was being depleted, steadily, with each additional demand that his system could not fully recover from overnight.

This is what borrowed capacity feels like from the inside. It feels like managing. It feels like coping. On the good days, it feels almost like health—a productive afternoon, a social engagement that went well, an evening that didn't cost the next morning. The cost of those good days is not felt until later: the crash that follows a productive week, the two days of recovery that a single social evening now requires, the way that an ordinary illness—a minor cold, a disrupted sleep schedule, or a stressful project at work, things a healthy system would absorb in a day or two—instead takes two weeks to recover from.

The borrowed capacity account does not send notices.

There is no warning when the balance is getting low. The first indication that the reserve has been exhausted is usually a worsening that seems disproportionate to its cause—a response to a minor stressor that is more severe and more prolonged than it should be. By that point, the borrowing has been going on for a long time.

What James's mitochondrial protocol did, in this context, was present a significant additional demand to a system that had no reserve left. In a system with reserve, this produces adaptation. In a system without reserve, it produces collapse.

Borrowed capacity is not a failure of character or an absence of resilience. It is what happens when the demands of life exceed what the body's physiology can currently sustain. The problem is that the borrowing is invisible until the account is empty—and by then, the person has often been told, by themselves and by others, that they are managing fine.

Reading Your Own History

Before we walk through the sequence layer by layer, I want to give you something for reading your own history through the lens of what we have discussed. Not a worksheet. A way of thinking about your own story that most patients have never been offered.

Think of the treatment that produced the strongest worsening. The one that cost you the most—the most time, the most hope, the most trust. Keep it in mind for a moment.

Now ask: what was that treatment aimed at? What layer of the sequence was it targeting? Was it a gut protocol? An energy intervention? A hormonal support protocol? An immune-modulating approach? Locate it in the map from Chapter 2. Find where it sits in the sequence.

Then ask: at the time you tried it, what was happening in the layers below it? How stable was your sleep—not just in hours, but in quality and restoration? How reactive was your nervous system—were you in a period of heightened sensitivity, or a period of relative calm? How much reserve did you actually have? Were you in a period of borrowed capacity, drawing on reserves that were already depleted, or were you in a period of genuine stability from which you had something to give?

Most patients who sit with these questions for a few minutes arrive at the same recognition: the layer below the treatment was not stable.

The sleep was disrupted. The nervous system was reactive. The reserve was low. The foundation that the treatment required in order to work had not been established. And the treatment—which was aimed at a real problem, correctly identified, and well-intentioned—arrived into a system that could not receive it.

That recognition is not a small thing. It changes the story from "my body cannot be helped" to "my body was not ready for that help at that time." Those are different stories. The first one closes doors. The second one reopens them.

You did not fail the treatment. The wrong sequence failed you. And that is something nobody explained to you until now.

There is a principle I share with my patients trying to make sense of a history like this:

When and how determine outcome more than what.

The specific treatment matters. But the timing of the treatment—and whether the body has the stability required to receive it—matters more. And the sequence in which treatments are applied ultimately determines whether the system can receive them or must reject them.

You were not failing to respond to treatment. Your body was telling you—precisely, consistently, and in the only language it has—that you were starting in the wrong place. And starting in the right place is entirely possible.

Foundation Work You Can Do Now

The practical tool for this chapter addresses the most foundational regulatory input available to the human body—one that predates every supplement, every pharmaceutical, every therapeutic protocol by hundreds of millions of years. It requires no equipment, no prescription, and no prior experience. It works at the level of the nervous system foundation, which means it is appropriate regardless of where you are in your history of illness.

The practice is slow, rhythmic breathing. Not breathing in the casual, vague sense that the word is often used in wellness contexts. A specific kind of breathing, with a specific physiologic target.

Here is what to do.

Find a place where you can lie down comfortably. A stable, supportive surface is usually ideal, but comfort comes first. The goal is to find a position you can maintain without unnecessary strain or distraction. Lie on your back and put your legs up—against a wall, against the couch, against anything stable. Your body should form a rough right angle at the hips, with your back flat and your legs elevated. If this is not comfortable or possible, lie flat.

Close your eyes. Let your arms rest at your sides, palms facing up. Give yourself a moment to let the position become familiar. If you need to make adjustments to become more comfortable, do so. The goal is not to force a position. The goal is to find one your body experiences as safe and comfortable enough to relax into.

Now breathe through your nose. In for four counts. Out for four counts. Nothing forced. Nothing dramatic. The breath should be quiet—so quiet that someone standing next to you might not notice you were doing anything at all. If four counts feels rushed, try five or six. The pace that feels completely natural to you, within that range, is the right pace for your system at this moment.

Do this for ten to fifteen minutes. Longer is better. But ten minutes, done consistently every day, will produce more benefit than thirty minutes done three times a week.

What is happening physiologically during this practice is precise and well-established. Slow, rhythmic nasal breathing at approximately five to six cycles per minute generates a phenomenon called respiratory sinus arrhythmia: a natural synchronization of your heart rate with your breathing cycle that is one of the most sensitive markers of a nervous system moving toward regulated function. Each breath in, the heart rate rises slightly. Each breath out, it falls. When this oscillation is smooth and consistent—which it becomes, with practice—it is a direct signal to the nervous system that the threat response can reduce its activity.

The legs-up position amplifies this. Elevating the legs reduces the circulatory demand on the heart, decreases the postural muscle activity that the nervous system is continuously monitoring, and creates a physiologic environment of reduced demand. The nervous system reads this environment and adjusts accordingly.

Together—the position and the breath—they send the clearest possible signal to a system that has been in protective mode: the demand is low. The immediate environment is safe. The alert can begin to reduce.

Here is what that shift feels like.

What you will notice first, if you do this consistently, is not dramatic. It is subtle—and that subtlety is worth paying attention to, because subtle is exactly what early progress feels like at this layer of recovery.

The shoulders drop. Not consciously—you didn't decide to lower them. They just release, on their own, as the autonomic system begins its shift. The jaw unclenches slightly. The chest, which in a chronically stressed system often carries a low-grade defensiveness—a bracing, a held quality—softens. The scanning that the nervous system does continuously—the background vigilance that most people with chronic illness have stopped noticing because it has been present so long—becomes slightly less insistent. The thoughts, which in a threatened state tend to move rapidly and repetitively, begin to slow.

Over days and weeks, the changes become more apparent. Sleep transitions become easier—not because you added another sleep supplement, but because the nervous system is less activated at the moment when sleep requires disengagement. Digestion becomes more predictable—not because anything changed in the gut directly, but because the autonomic signal that governs gut motility has shifted toward the parasympathetic state that digestion requires. The internal urgency—the background sense that something must be managed, addressed, monitored—begins to lose its constant pressure.

These are the early signs of a foundation beginning to stabilize. They are not proof of recovery. They are the beginning of the conditions under which recovery becomes possible.

Do it today. Do it tomorrow. Do it every day, and notice what changes.

Not dramatically, usually. But specifically. A morning that feels slightly less effortful. A night that gives slightly more back. A reaction to something that would normally set you back—a stressful exchange, an unexpected change in plans—that passes a little more quickly than it used to.

Small changes in the foundation produce large changes in everything above it.

James recovered. Not quickly, and not without difficulty. But the recovery was real, and it followed a sequence—the sequence that his system had been trying to tell him it needed all along.

He reassessed the promotion and took it. Not because the fear was entirely gone, but because the calculation he had been running for three years—the constant assessment of whether he had enough reserve to sustain one more demand—had finally quieted enough that he could hear something else. He told me later that the first morning he arrived at a new project without having pre-determined his exit strategy was the morning he understood what recovery actually felt like.

He came in about fourteen months after we began working together. He said that the experience of his illness—the two lost months, the failed protocol, the particular despair of a systematic thinker whose system had stopped working—had taught him something that nothing in his professional life had managed to teach him.

"I learned that some problems don't respond to better analysis," he said. "They respond to correct sequencing. The analysis was right. The sequence was wrong. It took me losing two months of my life to understand that. I had the right pieces; I was just reading the map backward."

And understanding the difference—understanding that the body's refusal to cooperate with a correct treatment is information about sequence rather than evidence of unfixability—is the beginning of finding the path that actually works.

In the next section of this book, we are going to walk through the sequence layer by layer. We will start at the foundation and work upward.

At each phase, we will look at what that phase does, what it requires from the one below it, and what the most common mistakes look like when a phase is misaddressed or skipped.

For now: the floor, the legs up, the breath. Four counts in. Four counts out. Ten minutes.

The foundation comes first.

CHAPTER FOUR

Safety First: The Nervous System Foundation

"Recovery begins when the nervous system no longer needs to continuously monitor, predict, defend against, or respond to excessive environmental demand. This is the most important phase to identify correctly. Everything else depends on getting this one right."
—Marcus Ettinger, DC

Some of the most difficult patients practitioners encounter are those whose nervous systems have become so sensitized that almost everything makes them worse. A new supplement provokes a reaction. A dietary change that helps most people triggers a flare. A gentle exercise protocol produces a crash. Even treatments specifically designed to calm the nervous system sometimes intensify it.

These patients often arrive having been told, implicitly or explicitly, that they are unusually sensitive—as if sensitivity were a personal trait rather than a physiologic state. Some have been told that their reactions are anxiety-driven, that the problem is psychological, and that if they could simply reduce their fear of symptoms they would stop having so many of them. A few have been told, with the damaging confidence of a practitioner who has run out of explanations, that they may just have to learn to live with it.

This presentation is known by many names. In this book, it is part of Phase 1, the Autonomic Foundation, and is referred to as Phase 1B, the sensitized autonomic state. It occurs when the nervous system has spent so long operating in threat mode that ordinary inputs begin to feel biologically threatening.

It is the most important presentation pattern in the entire sequence to identify correctly. Not the most dramatic. Not the most complex. The most important. Because a patient in this sensitized state who is treated as though they are in another phase will worsen on interventions aimed at that phase. The interventions are not wrong. The foundation required to receive them has not yet been established.

Not every patient presenting with reactivity and sensitivity is in this sensitized state. Some have isolated sensitivities with stable foundations. Some have overlapping presentations that require clinical differentiation. What this chapter describes is a recognizable pattern—one that appears across many patients with many different diagnoses—not an explanation for all reactivity. The framework interprets. It does not replace clinical judgment.

What is actually happening to patients in the sensitized autonomic state is the clearest possible expression of the sequence in action. They are not uniquely broken. They are not psychologically causing their own symptoms. They are living in a nervous system that has remained in a sustained threat response long enough to lower its sensitivity threshold so low that almost any input—physiologic, sensory, or chemical—registers as a potential danger.

The Game Face

Her name is Rachel. She was thirty-eight years old, a social media marketing manager, and she had walked into my office holding what she described as her game face—the same face she had been wearing through most of the last year and a half.

Thirteen years of marriage. One discovery. She moved out that same week. The divorce itself was still in process; the affair had not been. There had been no period of decline before any of this—no long history of unexplained symptoms, no slow deterioration. There had been a marriage that everyone, including Rachel, described as troubled but workable, and then a text she should not have looked at, and then everything that followed.

Four months after she moved out—she remembered the date because Breana had been at a sleepover that night—she woke with what she thought was a heart attack. Pounding chest, breath she could not catch, an alarm in her body so loud and so specific that she drove herself to urgent care at three in the morning. The EKG was normal. The bloodwork was normal. The physician told her that she was having a panic attack and should follow up with her primary care doctor about anxiety.

That had been the first one. Within weeks, she developed gastritis severe enough to make her afraid to eat. The palpitations returned. Headaches appeared without warning. Then came something harder to explain. The smell of perfume in an elevator. The fluorescent lights in a conference room. A crowded grocery store on a Saturday morning. A song coming on too loudly in the car. Things that had once been background noise now felt impossible to ignore.

"My body became a stranger that flinched at things," she said.

None of it made sense to her. She had assumed, in the way most people do, that her body would eventually adjust to the new shape of her life. Instead, it seemed to become less able to tolerate it.

What followed was not dramatic. It was gradual. And because it was gradual, almost nobody noticed.

The sensitivities did not stay where they started. The perfume in the elevator was only the beginning. Soon it was the deodorant of the man standing next to her, and the cleaning product used in the building lobby. The fluorescent lights in the conference room became the fluorescent lights in every overhead fixture in the office, then in the grocery store. Each input that her nervous system had once filtered without effort was now something it could no longer reliably filter.

The world had become difficult to tune out.

What she lost, in those months, was not a list of activities. It was the ability to predict how long she could stay anywhere before her body would tell her she had to leave.

A meeting that started fine could become unbearable forty minutes in. A grocery run on a Tuesday afternoon was manageable; the same store on a Saturday morning was not. She could not tell, walking into anything, whether this would be one of the times she could stay through it or one of the times she would have to find a reason to step outside.

Home was the only place where the variables held still. She had gradually rearranged her life around it—working from home when her job allowed, ordering groceries when she could afford to, declining what she could decline—because home was the only environment in which she could reasonably predict how her body would respond. The cost of being anywhere else was the cost of not knowing.

"The symptoms were bad," she told me. "But not trusting my own body was worse."

Breana had started doing the dishes after dinner. Rachel had not asked her to. A few months later she noticed that Breana had started doing the laundry too—folding it into neat stacks on the bed the same way Rachel used to. One evening Rachel walked into the room and found her working quietly by herself. She stood there for a moment without speaking. Then she thanked her, walked upstairs, turned on the bathroom faucet, and cried where nobody could hear.

"She's twelve," Rachel said. "She shouldn't be the one noticing what needs to be done."

She paused.

"I keep telling myself I just have to hold it together until things settle. Just keep my game face on. But something is happening to me and I don't understand what it is."

For the first time since the appointment began, her voice cracked.

"And I don't have time to fall apart."

That was as close as she got, during our first meeting, to letting the held thing slip.

What she feared more than feeling worse was becoming someone her daughter had to accommodate. Someone unreliable. Someone absent. Someone who was physically present but increasingly unavailable.

She placed her face in her hands.

You are not difficult. You are managing the unmanageable in a body whose limits nobody else can fully see.

That is what a sensitized autonomic state costs. Not just the symptoms. The life around the symptoms.

What the Nervous System Is Actually Doing

Your nervous system has one primary job that supersedes all others: keeping you alive. Everything else it does—regulating your heart rate, managing your digestion, coordinating your immune response, governing your sleep—is in service of that primary job. And when the nervous system perceives a sustained threat to survival, it reorganizes its priorities accordingly.

The reorganization is not subtle. The nervous system does not simply become more alert. It fundamentally changes the way it processes incoming information. The sensitivity threshold drops—meaning that inputs which would normally be filtered out as irrelevant or manageable now register as significant. The response amplitude increases—meaning that when the system does respond, it responds harder and faster than it would in a stable state. And the recovery time lengthens—meaning that once activated, the system takes longer to return to baseline before it begins to stabilize.

This is what is meant, clinically, by sensitization. The nervous system has recalibrated—specifically and purposefully—to maximize detection and response to an environment it has assessed as dangerous. In an acutely dangerous environment, this recalibration saves lives. It is one of the most effective protective adaptations in mammalian biology.

The problem is time. Acute danger is supposed to resolve. The threat appears, the system mobilizes, the threat passes, the system restores its baseline sensitivity and returns to the business of regulation and repair. It is the cycle the nervous system is designed to operate within.

When the physiologic burden accumulates faster than it can be resolved, the nervous system never receives a clear signal that the danger has ended. It does not return to baseline. It holds the recalibration. Over time, what was an appropriate emergency response becomes the resting state of the system.

The longer this state persists, the more the body adapts to it as its new normal. Tolerance for ordinary physiologic, sensory, and emotional demands drops. Signaling becomes distorted. Recovery capacity shrinks. A nervous system that has been in sustained threat mode for months may return to baseline relatively quickly once the foundation becomes stable again. A nervous system that has remained in that state for years has adapted much more deeply. It takes longer to come back, requires more careful sequencing, and requires patience with a timeline that is longer than anyone wants.

A nervous system that has been in sustained threat response long enough begins to interpret the absence of threat as suspicious rather than safe. It has forgotten, in a functional sense, what normal feels like. And in that state, almost anything can feel like a threat—including treatment.

Why the Right Treatment Makes It Worse: Signal Before Inhibition

There is a specific mechanism behind the phenomenon James described in Chapter 3—the experience of getting dramatically worse on treatments that should have helped. I call it Signal Before Inhibition.

In a healthy, well-regulated nervous system, every incoming signal—from a supplement, a food, an exercise session, a medication, an environmental input—passes through an inhibitory gate before it produces a systemic response. That gate is not a metaphor. It is a real neural function, maintained by specific inhibitory circuits in the central and peripheral nervous system, that evaluates incoming signals and modulates the response. Strong signal, appropriate response. Weak signal, filtered out. Borderline signal, dampened to manageable.

In the sensitized state, that gate is compromised. And what happens as a result is consistent and predictable: when a new input arrives—including an otherwise appropriate treatment—it does not pass through a functioning gate. It hits the system at full amplitude. There is nothing to modulate the response.

Because the nervous system has remained organized around threat, the circuits that normally dampen incoming signals are no longer functioning at full strength. Ordinary inputs arrive too loud. A conversation that should be manageable is overwhelming. A supplement taken at a fraction of the standard dose produces a reaction that feels wildly disproportionate to the dose itself. The filtering mechanism that a regulated system uses to decide what deserves a response and what can safely be ignored is not functioning. Everything gets through. Everything gets registered. The result is a persistent sense of being internally flooded—not by any single input, but by the accumulation of inputs the system cannot screen. This is why small things feel biologically enormous in the sensitized autonomic state.

A B-complex vitamin, introduced to support nerve function, increases neural signaling in a system that is already amplifying every signal it receives. The vitamin is not wrong. The system is not allergic to it. But the signaling increase that the vitamin produces has no functioning filter to moderate it. The system responds to the increase as though it were a threat. Symptoms worsen. A probiotic, containing live bacteria that will interact with the gut-immune barrier, generates an immune response that a regulated system would manage easily but that a sensitized system amplifies into a flare.

None of these treatments is wrong. None of these patients is uniquely sensitive in the personal sense.

What is wrong is the sequence. The nervous system's ability to moderate incoming signals must be restored before stimulating treatments can be tolerated. Because without that architecture, the signal has no functioning gate to pass through, and the system responds to every therapeutic input as though it were an alarm.

This is the clinical principle that changes how I approach every patient in a sensitized autonomic state. The question is not "what does this patient need?" The question is "what can this patient's system currently receive without triggering amplification?" And the answer, in the sensitized autonomic state, is: inputs that reduce the load rather than add to it. Inputs that communicate to the nervous system that the environment is manageable rather than threatening. Inputs that begin the slow, careful work of rebuilding the filtering architecture—not by targeting it directly, but by reducing the sustained threat signal that has been weakening it.

Rachel described this, when I explained it to her, as the first thing she had heard in the past year that made her own body make sense to her. Earlier in our conversation, she had mentioned that a magnesium supplement her primary care doctor recommended for anxiety had triggered three days of palpitations and insomnia.

"So when the magnesium made me worse," she said. "It wasn't that I'm broken."

"No," I said. "It was that the gate wasn't working. The magnesium sent a signal. The signal had nowhere to land softly. Your system amplified it. That's not a broken body. That's a body that's lost one specific function—the function of moderating incoming signals. And that function can be restored."

She was quiet for a moment.

"Can it actually be restored?" she asked. "After this long?"

"Yes," I said. "Because what changed was an adaptation—not permanent damage. Adaptations can be changed. More slowly than either of us would like. But yes."

When the Pattern Is More Complex: Two Amplifying Overlays

In some patients, the sensitized autonomic state is only part of the story. Two additional patterns can amplify autonomic reactivity, increase symptom intensity, and make stabilization more difficult. Neither one changes the fundamental treatment sequence—the foundation must still be established first. But understanding these patterns helps explain why some people experience this state more intensely than others, and why their path back to stability can take longer.

The first is the histamine and immune amplifier pattern. In a subset of patients in this sensitized state—particularly those with histories of allergies, asthma, eczema, food sensitivities across multiple categories, temperature dysregulation, or a strong reaction to fragrances and chemicals—there is an additional layer of immune reactivity operating alongside the nervous system sensitization. Certain immune cells, called mast cells, are primed to release inflammatory chemicals in response to a wide range of triggers: foods, environmental chemicals, stress, temperature changes, infections, and even certain medications. In a regulated system, mast cell activity is moderated by the same filtering mechanisms we discussed above. In a sensitized system, that modulation is reduced. The mast cells fire more readily, release more inflammatory chemicals, and the consequences—flushing, digestive disturbance, brain fog, joint pain, fatigue, and cardiovascular issues—layer on top of the existing sensitization.

The reactions often feel disproportionate and unpredictable. The same food that was fine last week causes a significant reaction this week. Cold temperatures trigger symptoms that seem unrelated to temperature. These patients often begin trying to identify every trigger. But the list keeps growing. They eliminate one food, then another, only to discover new reactions appearing where none existed before. The list never seems to stabilize.

This is not a separate diagnosis requiring a separate treatment track. It is the sensitized autonomic state with an immune amplifier.

The foundation work is the same.

What changes is the expectation of timeline—this pattern stabilizes more slowly—and the understanding that the apparent food sensitivities are not fixed allergies. They are reactivity patterns generated by a system that has lost its regulatory restraint, and they will reduce as the foundation stabilizes.

The second amplifying pattern appears predominantly in women and is rarely acknowledged, despite being clinically common. When the nervous system remains in a sustained threat response long enough, the normal regulation of reproductive hormones begins to change. The hormonal rhythm that governs the menstrual cycle becomes disrupted, and the result may be an elevation of androgens—testosterone and its metabolites. This pattern is not driven primarily by ovarian pathology. It is a downstream consequence of the sustained threat response.

For many women, this pattern shows up as irregular or worsened menstrual cycles, new or worsened adult acne, increased hair thinning, and sometimes the kind of emotional volatility and reactivity that gets attributed to anxiety or a mood disorder when it is actually another expression of the same underlying physiology.

Women with this pattern have often been told they have polycystic ovarian syndrome, or a hormonal imbalance that requires hormonal treatment. In some cases those diagnoses are correct. In many cases the pattern is a neuroendocrine expression of a sensitized autonomic state, and it resolves as the nervous system foundation stabilizes—usually without requiring direct hormonal intervention.

The important point is that these patterns change the intensity of the presentation, not the order of recovery. They can make the journey slower, more reactive, and more confusing. They do not change where healing begins. The foundation still comes first.

The Two Categories of Intervention

This brings us to one of the most important clinical distinctions in this book—one that is almost never made explicit in the patient's experience of treatment but determines everything about what will help and what will harm in the sensitized state.

Every treatment you might use in the process of recovering your health falls into one of two categories. The first is load-based treatments: things that require your system to process, adapt, and respond. Supplements. Medications. Dietary changes. Exercise protocols. Detoxification programs. These are not bad treatments—they are often the right treatments at the right time. But they are physiologically active. They add to the system's processing demand. And in a system that is already at its regulatory ceiling, adding demand—even with something theoretically beneficial—produces the results we discussed in Chapter 3: amplification, worsening, or no response.

The second category is safety-signal interventions: things that reduce the regulatory load rather than adding to it. Interventions that send the nervous system a clear signal that the immediate environment is not dangerous, that vigilance can temporarily decrease, that the inhibitory architecture can begin to rebuild. These interventions do not feel like treatment. They do not target a specific finding or correct a specific deficiency. They work at the level of the nervous system's fundamental assessment of the environment—and that assessment, as we have seen, is what determines whether everything else can work.

Safety-signal interventions are not supplemental. They are not the thing you do while waiting for the real treatment to work. In the sensitized state, they are the real treatment. They are what makes everything else possible.

What are safety-signal interventions? They include time in natural environments—not structured nature therapy, but simply being outside, in a green space, in relative quiet, without the demand of social performance or sensory overload. They include consistent, predictable daily routines—because predictability reduces the nervous system's need to continuously scan for change. They include the specific breathing practice described in Chapter 3. They include reducing sensory input in the home environment—dimmer lighting, lower ambient noise, fewer demands on attention. They include gentle movement that does not push past the threshold of physiologic challenge.

None of these sound like medicine. That is the point. The sensitized nervous system is not responsive to medicine in the conventional sense—not yet. It is responsive to the message that the environment is safe. And once that signal begins to register, the threshold begins to rise. The inhibitory architecture begins to rebuild. The system begins to recover the regulatory capacity it has been spending on continuous vigilance. And with that capacity restored, even incrementally, the treatments that could not previously be tolerated begin to become tolerable.

The Amplification Paradox

There is a specific phenomenon in the sensitized state that accounts for much of the confusion—and much of the self-blame—that people experience during recovery.

In a sensitized nervous system, physiologic amplification is not proportional to the size of the input. A small input can produce a large response. A supplement taken at a fraction of the standard dose can produce a reaction that looks, to both the patient and the practitioner, like a severe adverse event. A twenty-minute walk can produce the kind of fatigue that would normally follow a full athletic competition. A minor stressor—a difficult conversation, a change in plans, a poor night's sleep—can destabilize the system for days.

The amplification is real. The response is not imagined or exaggerated. But it is not proportional in the normal sense, and that disproportionality is what makes it so confusing. The patient knows, rationally, that a twenty-minute walk should not produce two days of exhaustion. The gap between what the body is doing and what it should be doing—by any reasonable standard—is the gap that produces shame. The assumption that something uniquely and permanently wrong explains it. The slow withdrawal from activities, relationships, and plans, because the cost has become too unpredictable to risk.

What has actually gone wrong is the calibration. The inhibitory architecture has been compromised. The nervous system is amplifying because amplification is what it has been set to do. Both the low threshold and the amplified response are features of the sensitized state, not bugs. They are doing exactly what they are supposed to do in a system that has assessed its environment as dangerous.

The clinical implication is this: when a patient in the sensitized state reports that a treatment made them dramatically worse, the information that report contains is not "this patient cannot tolerate this treatment." It is "this patient's nervous system is currently amplifying all inputs, including this treatment, because the inhibitory gate is not functioning." The appropriate response is not to conclude that the treatment is wrong or that the patient is uniquely broken. It is to recognize that the inhibitory architecture must be restored before load-based interventions can be received.

Rachel, once she understood this, sat quietly for a moment. Then she said something I have thought about many times since.

"I've been blaming myself for over a year," she said. "Every time something made me worse, I thought I was the problem. That I was doing something wrong. That my body had decided to be unfixable."

She looked at her hands.

"It wasn't me. It was the sequence."

"It was the sequence," I said.

Widening the Margin

A question I hear a lot from patients in a sensitized autonomic state is: I understand that I need to stabilize before I advance. But what does stabilizing actually look like? What am I trying to build toward, and how do I know when I've gotten there?

The goal of this work is the widening of the margin—the gradual expansion of what the system can absorb without cascading. Someone in a sensitized autonomic state may not be able to tolerate a new supplement, a disrupted sleep schedule, a busy social week, or an unfamiliar food without significant consequence. As stability returns, those variations become increasingly manageable. That is the difference between restricted stability and true stability, which we discussed in Chapter 2. The margin has widened enough that ordinary life fits inside it.

The process of widening that margin follows a sequence of its own. It begins not with adding inputs but with reducing load—the safety-signal work we have been discussing. The breathing practice. The consistent schedule. The time in natural environments. The reduction of unnecessary sensory demand. These do not directly expand the margin. They reduce the demand of maintaining a defensive posture, allowing regulatory capacity to recover.

The next step is the careful, incremental introduction of variation—not therapeutic inputs, but ordinary life variations that the system needs to learn to tolerate. A slightly different meal composition. A slightly longer social engagement. A modest change in the daily schedule. Each variation, introduced at a level that is just at the edge of what the system can currently absorb without destabilizing, trains the inhibitory architecture to manage that level of input. The system learns, through repeated tolerated exposure, that the input is not dangerous. The threshold for that input rises. The margin widens slightly.

A system that has been in sustained sensitization for years does not recalibrate in weeks. The nervous system requires repetition—many experiences of being exposed to a variation and surviving it without consequence—before it will update its threat assessment for that variation. Rushing the process, introducing variations that exceed the current margin, produces the amplification response rather than the recalibration response. The margin does not widen. It contracts.

Most patients in this phase misread stabilization. They expect recovery to feel like something—a lift, a lightness, a return of energy that announces itself. What they get instead is subtraction: a crash that lasted one day instead of three, a stressful conversation that passes in an evening, a food that causes mild discomfort instead of a multi-day reaction. These subtractions are easy to dismiss because they feel like slightly less bad rather than dramatically better. But slightly less bad, sustained consistently across weeks, is the nervous system recalibrating. The margin is widening. The system is not better yet, but it is becoming more capable of holding ordinary life without losing its footing. That is the work.

Rachel described the first sign of it as noticing that she had been sitting in traffic for fifteen minutes without calculating how much longer she could tolerate it before she had to pull off. Not without registering the traffic—she registered it. But the calculation had stopped being the first thing her mind did when the cars slowed. The margin was widening. She had not felt it. She had simply noticed, afterward, that one of the calculations had been running less urgently than before.

What I tell patients in this phase is: measure progress by what the system can absorb, not by how it feels.

Foundation Work You Can Do Now

By now, the pattern should be becoming clear. A sensitized nervous system recovers through repeated experiences that allow it to lower its guard. The practice for this chapter is deceptively simple. It creates the conditions in which that process can occur.

Here is what is actually happening when a sensitized nervous system is placed in a natural environment.

The human nervous system evolved over hundreds of thousands of years in natural environments. The sensory profile of those environments—the specific frequencies of light filtered through leaves, the irregular rhythms of wind and water, the absence of the sharp, unpredictable sensory events that characterize human-built environments—is, at a neurological level, familiar in a way that modern environments are not. The brain processes natural sensory input with lower cognitive and autonomic load than it processes urban or indoor sensory input. The nervous system can begin to reduce its vigilance because the environment contains fewer rapid, unpredictable changes that the threat-detection system has evolved to detect.

Research has quantified these effects with enough precision that they are no longer matters of opinion or personal experience. Time in natural environments measurably reduces activity within the amygdala—one of the brain's primary threat-detection regions. It is also associated with lower cortisol, improvements in heart rate variability, and reductions in markers of inflammation.

These effects begin within minutes and accumulate with consistent exposure.

Nature is not simply the absence of urban stress. It appears to provide a distinct biologic signal that shifts the brain toward a less threat-oriented state.

For the sensitized nervous system, this makes natural environments uniquely valuable—not as a nice extra, but as a specific therapeutic input aimed at the foundational layer of the sequence. It reduces load. It communicates safety. It gives the inhibitory architecture the opportunity to begin rebuilding.

Here is the practice.

Once each day, go outside into a natural or semi-natural environment—a park, a garden, a tree-lined street, a patch of grass, a body of water. It does not need to be wilderness. It does not need to be beautiful. It needs to be outside, and it needs to have some element of the natural world present.

Do not bring your phone to look at. Do not bring a podcast. Do not bring a task to accomplish. Bring only yourself, and for ten to twenty minutes, simply be present in the environment. Walk slowly if you want to walk. Sit if you want to sit. The goal is not exercise and it is not mindfulness in the structured sense of the word. The goal is to allow your nervous system to be in an environment it is neurologically predisposed to experience as lower-threat.

If you are in a sensitized state, start with ten minutes. Starting shorter than you think you need to is always safer than starting longer. The nervous system in this state does not benefit from being pushed—it benefits from being given inputs it can process without triggering amplification. Ten minutes of genuine physiologic ease is more restorative than thirty minutes of forced exposure that tips into overwhelm.

Do this every day. Not most days. Every day. The nervous system learns through repetition—through repeated exposure to the same lower-threat environment and the experience of moving through it without consequence. Consistency is what allows the signal to accumulate into a lasting shift in baseline calibration.

Combine this with the breathing practice from Chapter 3. Do the breathing before you go outside if the sensitized state makes outdoor environments feel activating rather than calming. Five or ten minutes of slow rhythmic breathing before nature exposure primes the nervous system toward the parasympathetic state and makes the natural environment more accessible as a safety signal.

These two practices—the breathing and the daily nature exposure—are the foundation of the foundation. They do not require a prescription. They do not add to the physiologic budget. They are safety-signal interventions: inputs that send the nervous system the environmental cue it needs to begin the process of recalibration.

You are not trying to push through the sensitized state. You are creating the conditions under which the nervous system chooses, on its own terms, to lower its guard. That distinction is everything.

Rachel recovered. Not quickly. The sensitized state takes time to recalibrate, and patience with that timeline is not optional. But the recovery was real, and it began the moment she stopped adding to the physiologic load and started, instead, reducing it.

She told me, about eight months into the process, that she had gone to one of Breana's cheerleading practices and sat on a bench at the edge of the field for the full hour. Other mothers were there. The noise was there. The unpredictability was there. Nothing happened. Her nervous system had not amplified. The alarm had not gone off.

"It was just a practice," she said. "Just an hour on a bench. But it felt like the first time in over a year that my body didn't treat the world like an emergency."

That is what recalibration feels like. Just an hour at her daughter's practice in which a bench was a bench, and the world did not feel like a threat.

And it is the beginning of everything.

In the next chapter, we will look at what becomes possible once the foundation stabilizes—the restoration of autonomic flexibility, the return of resilience, and the specific patterns that tell you the nervous system is beginning to operate from safety rather than sustained alert.

CHAPTER FIVE

The Regulation Gate: When Calm Becomes Possible

Regulation is not how little a system reacts.
It is how reliably it returns.
—Marcus Ettinger, DC

The most important turning point in recovery is not the dramatic one people imagine when they think of getting better. It is an easily-missed shift that often first becomes clear in a conversation I have with patients.

The patient comes in for a follow-up appointment. They sit down. I ask how things have been. And they say, with a tone of hedged optimism that tells me they have been disappointed before: "I think things might be a little better. But I'm not sure."

I ask them what "a little better" means to them.

They think about it. "My coworker wore strong perfume in the office on Wednesday. A few months ago that would have given me a headache that lasted into the next day. This time I noticed it, and that was it. It was just a smell." Or: "I had a tense call with my sister on Sunday morning. I expected it to wreck me for the rest of the day—it always does. But by lunch I felt pretty normal. I kept waiting for the crash. It didn't come." Or: "I slept five nights in a row without waking up at two in the morning. I can't remember the last time that happened."

These are not dramatic recoveries. They are not the improvements that shows up on a lab panel or a practitioner's notes. But they are the signs I look for most carefully, because they tell me something specific and important: the foundation is beginning to hold. The nervous system is beginning to do what it has not been able to do reliably for a very long time: activate when it needs to, and return to baseline when it doesn't. The alarm is beginning to quiet down.

This is what the end of Phase 1 looks like.

It's not the complete disappearance of symptoms. It's not a return to who the patient was before they got sick, and it's not a single dramatic moment of arrival. It is the point at which the foundation has become strong enough to support everything that comes next.

The last chapter described how Phase 1 begins. This chapter is about recognizing the moment the regulation gate begins to open—when the nervous system no longer has to devote all of its resources to reacting and can finally begin supporting repair, adaptation, and resilience.

What regulation looks like in everyday life. How to know when the foundation has held. And how to recognize the difference between fragile stability and genuine resilience.

What Regulation Actually Means

The word "regulation" is used so broadly in health and wellness that its clinical meaning has become blurred. I want to use it here with a much more specific definition, because that definition is what matters clinically.

In this book, regulation is defined by how reliably the nervous system returns to baseline after it reacts.

A regulated nervous system is not necessarily a calm one. It is a flexible one. It is a system that can shift appropriately in response to demand—activating when it needs to and returning to baseline when it doesn't.

The key word is return.

The capacity to return to baseline after a challenge is what distinguishes a regulated system from a sensitized one.

Think of it as the difference between a thermostat that works and one that is stuck. A functioning thermostat responds when the temperature moves away from the set point. It activates the heating or cooling system as needed and turns it off once the set point is reached again. A stuck thermostat either fails to respond to deviations or, more commonly in the clinical picture of chronic illness, responds to every deviation with maximum force and then fails to turn off.

In the sensitized state, the nervous system is the stuck thermostat. It activates—to stress, to sensory input, to a new supplement, to a difficult conversation—with more force than the situation warrants, and it takes longer than it should to return to its resting state. Every cycle of activation that does not fully resolve before the next one arrives leaves the system slightly further from baseline. Over time, this accumulation of unresolved activation cycles becomes the resting state itself.

Regulation—the restoration of autonomic flexibility—is the process by which the system learns to work again. Not to stop responding to challenges, but to respond proportionally and, crucially, to recover from them. The return to baseline after activation is the clinical marker I am looking for. It is what "a little better" actually means.

This distinction matters more than it might appear. Many patients—and many practitioners—conflate regulation with calmness. They interpret the goal of this phase as achieving a state in which the patient no longer reacts to things. That is not the goal. A nervous system that has been pharmaceutically sedated into non-reactivity is not regulated. It is suppressed. And suppression, while sometimes necessary in the short term, does not produce the recovery of function that genuine regulation does.

The goal is not a nervous system that does not react. It is a nervous system that reacts proportionally and recovers reliably.

When a system can activate and return to baseline, it has begun to move through the regulation gate. What lies beyond is not perfect health, but the possibility of sustained recovery.

The Gate

I call this layer of the hierarchy the regulation gate, and the name is deliberate. A gate is not a destination. It is a threshold—a point that must be passed before the next territory becomes accessible. You do not stay at the gate. But you cannot bypass it, and you cannot pretend you have passed through it when you haven't.

The regulation gate is the point at which the nervous system has become stable enough that it can tolerate mild variation without losing its footing. Where a supplement introduced at a low dose no longer triggers a full-system alarm. Where a slightly busier day does not require three days of recovery. Where sleep, though still imperfect, is becoming more consistent. Where the patient can report that things are a little better.

The gate matters because of what it makes possible above it. As long as the nervous system remains in a highly sensitized state, the immune system cannot regulate. It is receiving a continuous signal from the nervous system that the environment is dangerous, and it responds to that signal by staying activated—generating inflammatory signals, keeping immune cells primed, maintaining a baseline of reactivity that ensures the gut remains irritable, the sinuses remain inflamed, the joints remain sore.

The immune system remains activated not because an active pathogen is necessarily present, but because the regulatory signals arriving from the foundation continue communicating that the environment is unsafe. When the nervous system begins to restabilize—when it crosses the regulation gate and regains the ability to return to baseline—the immune system receives a different signal. The downstream inflammatory response begins to diminish. The gut begins to calm. The food reactions that felt like fixed allergies begin to lessen. And the layer above the immune system—the circadian system—begins to re-establish the patterns that allow sleep to become more restorative, energy more predictable, and recovery more reliable.

None of this happens dramatically. It happens in the same way that the patient in the earlier follow-up appointment described.

A few good days. A reaction that passes faster than before. A night of sleep that felt, for once, actually restorative. These are not coincidences.

They are the early signs of a sequence beginning to self-correct from the foundation upward.

The gate also has a consequence when it is bypassed.

Understanding the regulation gate also explains why so many well-designed treatments appear to fail. Treatment failure often begins when a practitioner or patient, seeing early improvement, increases the system's load before the foundation is ready. That could mean moving from Phase 1 into Phase 2 too early, or adding a new intervention before the system has developed the capacity to receive it.

The pattern is predictable. Phase 2 treatments—gut protocols, antimicrobial support, barrier repair work—are introduced. The immune system, still receiving an intermittent regulatory signal from an incompletely stabilized nervous system, interprets the additional physiologic inputs as threat rather than support. Inflammatory signaling increases. Symptoms that had been quieting begin to return. The patient and practitioner conclude that Phase 2 therapy was the wrong approach, discontinue it, and return to baseline—sometimes below it.

The problem was not Phase 2 therapy. The problem was timing. The nervous system was not yet stable enough to allow the immune system to receive the treatment without amplifying it. The gate had not been passed.

The consequence of trying to build above a foundation that has not yet stabilized is always the same: the structure does not hold.

Maria

Her name is Maria. She was forty-four years old, a graphic designer who worked from home. She came to me as a new patient after six years managing a body that required constant negotiation. She wasn't there because she had recently become worse. She had begun to suspect that the management itself had become the problem.

She was not sensitized in the way Rachel had been. She did not react dramatically to ordinary inputs. She did not have panic episodes. She had no acute onset she could point to, no inflection moment that had broken her body. What she had was something more subtle: a foundation that had been functioning, for years, just well enough to keep her life intact and just poorly enough to require her to engineer everything around it.

"I'm not sick in a way anyone would recognize," she told me. "I can get up. I can work. I can do most of what I need to do. I'm just always one thing away from not being able to."

That phrase—one thing away—is worth sitting with. It captures something that most people with chronic illness recognize immediately but that is almost impossible to convey to someone who has not lived it. It is not the experience of being unwell. It is the experience of being perpetually on the edge of being unwell. And it is the clinical signature of a patient whose nervous system has stabilized partially but has never crossed the threshold that would allow it to absorb ordinary variation without cascading.

When stability depends on conditions being perfect, ordinary life becomes a continuous negotiation. One bad night changes the week. One stressful phone call changes digestion for the rest of the day. One skipped meal changes sleep. One social event changes the three days that follow. The system is functioning—but only inside tightly controlled parameters, and the effort required to maintain those parameters is invisible to everyone except the person doing it. This is not dramatic collapse. It is fragility. And fragility, sustained across years, trains a person to calculate costs that everyone else spends without thinking.

Maria had not stopped doing things in the obvious way that Rachel had in Chapter 4. She had not withdrawn from events or stopped going to restaurants. She had found ways to go to the restaurant—but she ate from a narrow, safe menu, sat near the exit, kept the visit short, and went home to rest before the evening was over. She attended her daughter's events—but she managed her energy in the week beforehand, declined the social engagements around them, and spent the following day in recovery. She accepted client work—but she had reduced her rates to allow more time per project, because the pace she had maintained five years ago was no longer available to her.

From the outside, this looked like a person who was functioning normally. From the inside, it was a daily calibration so practiced that she no longer noticed she was performing it. Every moment of apparent normalcy was purchased at a cost that did not appear on any ledger but was paid, reliably, in the hours and days that followed.

She had tried, over the years, to address specific aspects of her condition—gut protocols, adrenal and thyroid support, and mitochondrial supplements. Each had produced some benefit; none of the benefits had held. She would feel better for a few weeks, sometimes a few months, and then something would happen—a stressful period, a minor illness, a disruption to her routine—and she would return to her previous baseline or below it.

"I keep getting close to feeling normal," she said. "And then I lose it. I can't tell if I'm doing something wrong or if this is just what my body is now."

What Maria was describing was not a problem with the treatments. It was a problem with the layer they were aimed at. Each targeted a layer above a foundation that remained incompletely stable. The autonomic system underneath was stable enough to allow some response to each treatment, but not stable enough to hold the response when ordinary life resumed. Every time, the foundation gave way under stress, and everything built on top of it gave way with it.

What Maria needed was not better treatments for her specific findings. She needed the regulation gate to close behind her—for the foundation to develop sufficient flexibility that ordinary life disruptions no longer consumed the entirety of her available reserve. She needed the foundation to hold.

How to Know If You Have Passed the Gate

The question is always the same: how do I know when I'm ready to move forward? How do I know that the foundation has held?

The honest answer is that it is not a single moment. It is a pattern that becomes visible over time, across four specific dimensions. It's not a formal assessment, but a set of observations that a patient can make about daily life.

The first dimension is response to dietary variation. Can you eat something outside your established safe list without predictable, significant consequence? Not without any consequence—some variation in response to dietary change is normal. But the response should be modest and short-lived, not the kind of multi-day reaction that characterized the sensitized state. If a slightly different meal produces a significantly different outcome every time, the foundation is not yet stable enough to support the immune work that comes next.

The second dimension is response to schedule disruption. When the routine is interrupted—a disrupted night's sleep, a changed work schedule, an unexpected demand—does the system recover within twenty-four to forty-eight hours? Or does a single disruption cascade into multiple days of destabilization? A regulated system can absorb variation and return to baseline. A system that is still at the gate cannot reliably do this yet.

The third dimension is stress recovery time. When something genuinely stressful occurs—a difficult interaction, unexpected bad news, a period of sustained pressure—how long does it take for the system to return to its stable baseline? In a regulated system, the recovery is proportional to the stressor and measured in hours or a day or two. In a system still at the gate, a significant stressor can produce a physiologic response that lasts for days, sometimes a week or longer.

The fourth dimension is the dependence on routine for stability. This is the most revealing question. If the three anchors introduced later in this chapter—wake time, meal rhythm, and wind-down—are held consistently, does the system feel relatively stable? And if they are disrupted for two or three days, does the system destabilize significantly? A system that requires perfect routine to maintain stability is in restricted stability—the gate has not yet been passed. A system that can absorb two or three days of routine disruption without cascading has developed the genuine regulatory flexibility that the next phase requires.

That is what transforms restricted stability into true stability. Stability no longer depends on avoiding disruption. It depends on the system's growing ability to return to baseline after disruption.

The regulation gate is not a moment. It is a pattern. And the pattern is this: the system can encounter variation and return to baseline, more than once, across more than one domain, consistently enough that the return—not the encounter—has become the expected outcome.

Why Progress Feels Like Nothing

One of the most clinically important things I can tell you about this layer of recovery is that the progress, when it comes, may not feel like progress. Not at first. It will not announce itself as recovery.

The experience of recovery in the regulation gate is not "I feel better." It is "I notice I reacted to that and then it passed." It is "I had a difficult week and I'm not as wrecked as I would have been six months ago." It is "I tried that food again and I was fine." These are subtractions—things that used to happen that no longer happen, or happen less severely, or pass more quickly.

There is a reason this kind of progress is so consistently missed. The nervous system is built to notice threat, intensity, and worsening. Pain announces itself. A crash registers immediately. A bad week is impossible to overlook. But normalization—the absence of something that used to happen, the softening of a reaction that used to be severe—does not trigger the same alert. The thing the patient has been bracing for never happens. And the human mind is poorly equipped to notice the absence of something it expected.

Recovery at this layer is not something the patient feels happening. It is something the patient notices in the things that no longer happen. The nervous system has been running in a state of continuous monitoring for so long that the monitoring no longer registers as a state—it registers as the patient's normal way of being. When the monitoring begins to ease, the patient often does not perceive the change as recovery. They notice that the body occupies less of their awareness than it once did.

This is why patients in the regulation gate often struggle to answer a simple question: "Are you better?" The improvements are real, but they are diffuse. The person notices they are thinking about symptoms less often. Less concerned about disruptions. Less aware of the body every moment of the day. The nervous system no longer dominates attention in the way it once did. And because the improvement is experienced as less interruption rather than more sensation, it can feel strangely difficult to measure—even while life itself is quietly becoming more livable.

The nervous system does not always reveal its learning in real time. Sometimes it practices a new pattern quietly before that pattern becomes visible. Recovery can feel repetitive long before it feels transformative. What feels like stagnation is often the nervous system rehearsing a different way of operating.

This phase of recovery is where patients are most at risk of losing faith in the process. The reason is easy to understand. The alternative—the load-based treatments that produce clear, dramatic, immediate effects, even if those effects don't hold—feels more like something is happening. More like treatment. More like progress. And the quiet, gradual widening of the regulatory margin, which is the real work of this phase, feels like very little.

I tell patients in this phase: do not measure progress by how you feel on a given day. Measure it by what your week contains. A week in which you reacted to something and recovered in hours rather than days is a week of real progress. A week in which you participated in something that, six months ago, you would have declined, is a week of real progress. A week in which you noticed the body less often than the week before is a week of real progress. The system is not better yet. But it is becoming more capable of participating in a normal life.

That capacity—the ability to absorb variation without cascading into dysfunction—is what resilience actually is. The system does not stop being challenged. It stops being undone by challenge. And it is the clinical marker that tells me the regulation gate has been passed and the sequence is ready for the next layer.

The body does not announce recovery. It demonstrates it in the things that no longer derail it. Learning to read those signs—rather than waiting for a dramatic announcement of wellness—is one of the most important skills in the process of healing.

The Consistency Principle

The single most important therapeutic variable at this layer of the sequence is one that feels so undramatic that most people underestimate it: consistency.

If there is one place patients are most likely to sabotage their own recovery, it is here. Consistency feels too simple to matter, so it is often the first thing they relax when they begin to feel a little better. In my experience, that single decision has delayed more recoveries than almost any supplement choice or treatment strategy.

The kind of consistency that matters most at this stage has very little to do with supplements. It has to do with the environment the nervous system experiences every day: the consistency of daily schedule, daily rhythm, and daily environmental inputs. Wake time. Meal times. Sleep time. The predictability of the day's structure.

Here is why this matters at a physiologic level. The nervous system is a pattern-recognition system. It is continuously scanning the environment—internal and external—for information about what to expect. When the environment is predictable, the scanning workload decreases. The nervous system does not need to generate and evaluate as many hypotheses about what might be coming next, because it already has a reliable model. That reduction in workload is a direct reduction in the regulatory burden—an increase in available capacity that can be redirected toward recovery and repair.

When the schedule is unpredictable, the body never fully settles. The system keeps waiting for the next interruption. Each variation—a meal that arrives late, a sleep schedule that shifts, a day that runs differently than expected—requires the nervous system to update its model of what is happening. Over time, that continuous updating becomes its own form of load. Vigilance becomes the baseline. The nervous system stops trusting the environment, because the environment has stopped being trustworthy.

And a nervous system that cannot trust the environment cannot invest in repair.

This is why the consistency of daily routine is not merely a helpful lifestyle recommendation at this layer. It is a direct physiologic intervention. Every morning you wake at the same time, your nervous system's prediction of the day becomes slightly more reliable. Every meal that arrives at a consistent time reduces the digestive system's need to be on continuous alert for intake. Every evening that follows a predictable pattern of reducing stimulation gives the circadian system the timing cues it needs to begin the transition toward sleep.

Predictability is, for the nervous system at the regulation gate, what safety signals are for the fully sensitized system. It is the input that communicates: the environment is manageable. You do not need to remain at maximum alert. You can begin to restore.

Foundation Work You Can Do Now

The practice for this chapter builds on the two practices from Chapters 3 and 4—the breathing and the nature exposure—and adds the third foundational pillar of nervous system recalibration: predictability. Predictability is the pillar. The three daily anchors are the practices that establish it.

Choose three times. One set wake time. One approximate meal timing pattern—it does not need to be to the minute, but it does need to be consistent within about an hour each day. And one set wind-down time—the time at which you begin the process of reducing stimulation in the evening, lowering lights, stepping away from screens and demanding cognitive activity, and allowing the body to begin its transition toward sleep.

These three anchors are not a sleep protocol or a diet. They are nervous system inputs—timing signals that the brain uses to predict, prepare for, and coordinate the daily cascade of physiologic events that constitutes regulated function. Every day you maintain these anchors, the nervous system's prediction of the day becomes slightly more reliable. And the more reliable the prediction, the less the system needs to remain on alert for what might come next.

If you are already keeping a consistent wake time from Chapter 2, you have the first anchor. Now add the second and third.

Here is what the wind-down anchor looks like in practice. At least sixty minutes before your target sleep time, begin reducing light in your home—dim the overhead lights, turn off screens or switch them to the warmest available color temperature, reduce ambient noise. Do not use this time for demanding work, difficult conversations, or anything that requires sustained attention and problem-solving. Use it for quiet, low-stimulation activity—reading something gentle, a relaxed conversation, slow movement, or the breathing practice from Chapter 3.

The physiology of this is direct. Your brain produces melatonin—the hormone that begins the transition into sleep—in response to darkness. Not total darkness, but a meaningful reduction in light relative to the daytime environment. When light exposure continues at full indoor intensity until the moment you try to sleep, the melatonin signal is suppressed and the transition is delayed.

When you begin reducing light an hour before sleep, the melatonin signal can rise in response to the changing light environment. As the melatonin signal rises, the nervous system begins transitioning into a state of reduced environmental monitoring that allows entry into sleep.

This is the evening disengagement process—the brain's gradual reduction of how much it is tracking and responding to the world around it. It is not something you can force. You cannot decide to disengage. You can only create the conditions under which disengagement becomes possible. Reduced light is one of those conditions. Reduced stimulation is another. Predictable timing—so the brain learns, through repeated patterns, to anticipate that this is the time disengagement begins—is the third.

Together, the three anchors—wake time, meal rhythm, wind-down—create a daily scaffold of predictability that the nervous system can use to reduce its vigilance load. They establish the conditions that allow the next layers of recovery to become accessible and, eventually, to hold.

One note on adherence: consistency matters more than perfection here, as it does in every practice in this book. A disrupted week does not erase the gains of a consistent month. The nervous system responds to the overall pattern, not to individual days. When the anchors drift, return to them without self-recrimination. The returning is part of the practice.

Maria began with these three anchors. She was skeptical—in the way that precise, analytical people are skeptical of interventions that seem too simple for the complexity of their problem. She had tried many things. Routine did not seem like a clinical intervention.

Eight weeks later, she reported something she had not experienced in years: three consecutive weeks without a single multi-day crash. Life had not been easy during those three weeks. There had been a difficult client situation, a family obligation that disrupted her schedule for a weekend, a minor illness that passed in four days. Any one of those, six months earlier, would have set her back significantly.

For the first time in years, she no longer felt as though ordinary life required negotiation every hour of the day.

"I don't know if this is the routine," she said, "or something else. But something is different."

It was the routine. Not in isolation—the breathing and the nature exposure had been building a foundation for weeks before the routine was added. But the routine was the intervention that widened the gate. That transformed restricted stability into true stability. That gave the nervous system enough consistent, predictable signals to trust the environment again.

She told me, about a month after that appointment, that she had accepted a client dinner—the first one in two years. Not because the calculation had disappeared. But because on that particular Tuesday, she had simply said yes before running the calculation. The calculation was still available. She just hadn't needed it yet.

That moment—saying yes before the calculation ran—is what it looks like when the foundation has become stable enough to support ordinary life again. The calculation had not disappeared. She could still have used it if she needed to. But for the first time in years, participation came before protection rather than after it.

The foundation has stabilized enough to support what comes next when ordinary life no longer requires continuous negotiation simply to absorb it.

This is the regulation gate. Not a destination. A threshold the foundation passes through, after which the next layer of recovery becomes accessible.

The next layer is the immune system—the conversation it has been having, all along, with the gut, the brain, and the body's inflammatory signaling network. That conversation has been distorted, for as long as the foundation has been incomplete, by the regulatory signal coming from below. As the foundation stabilizes, the immune system begins to receive a different signal. The conversation begins to change. The food reactions that felt like fixed allergies begin to ease. The gut, which has been irritable for reasons that were never primarily about the gut, begins to settle.

That is the work of Phase 2. And it can begin, now, because the foundation underneath it has held.

CHAPTER SIX

The Immune Conversation

"The gut does not fail in isolation.
It responds to the conditions surrounding it.
Change the conditions.
Everything else follows."
—Marcus Ettinger, DC

Sophie

Her name is Sophie. She was thirty-six years old and had been a nurse for eleven years when she first came to see me—a career she had chosen partly out of genuine vocation and partly because she had always wanted to understand how the body worked. She had that understanding. It had not helped her.

She had been managing food reactions for nine years. The reactions were not classic allergies—her IgE testing had been negative twice, which was one of the first sources of confusion, because the responses she experienced were real and reproducible and sometimes severe. Bloating. Cramping. A full-body inflammatory response that included joint pain, skin flushing, and brain fog that could last for several days. She had learned, through years of trial and error as well as careful observation, which foods were reliably safe and which reliably triggered symptoms. The list of safe foods had been shrinking for three years.

She did not describe this the way patients without clinical training describe it. She described it the way a nurse describes a patient's case—sys tematically, with the specific vocabulary of someone who had looked up every mechanism and still could not explain what was happening to her. She knew about barrier permeability. She knew about immune tolerance. She knew about the microbiome's role in gut health. She had read the research. None of it told her why her safe food list kept contracting despite everything she was doing correctly.

"I understand enough physiology to know that my body is reacting for a reason," she told me. "What I don't understand is why the reasons keep changing."

That was the precise description of her situation. The reactions were not random—they followed patterns she could partially identify—but the patterns shifted. A food that had been safe for months would suddenly become a trigger. A trigger she had carefully avoided for a year would occasionally be tolerable. The rules she had built her diet around kept failing her, and each failure required building new rules, which required more restriction, which left her eating from an increasingly narrow list while privately wondering how much narrower it could become before the shrinking list began creating problems of its own.

What had begun as dietary awareness had gradually become environmental management. She no longer ate spontaneously. Social invitations, travel, long workdays, even routine errands were filtered through the calculation of what she would eat and whether it would be safe. She carried food with her in a way that had become so routine she barely noticed it: snacks in her bag, a safe meal in her car on longer days, a mental inventory of what was available in any space she entered.

She had begun, without deciding to, scanning environments for exits and options before she fully committed to being in them. Travel had become something she declined more often than she accepted, not because she did not want to go but because the planning required to make travel safe had become more exhausting than staying home. The fear was not of the food itself. It was of being somewhere unfamiliar, without options, when the body decided to respond.

The reactions themselves were only part of the burden. The larger burden was the amount of life that had to be organized around preventing them.

At work, she managed the problem invisibly. She brought her own food to every shift, declining invitations to staff lunches and work dinners with explanations that felt close enough to true—she was watching her diet, she had some sensitivities, nothing serious. She had stopped going to the monthly birthday lunches in her unit, not because she did not want to go, but because restaurants required a level of food negotiation that was exhausting to perform in a social context while also pretending it was not happening. More often than she would have chosen, she ate lunch alone in her car.

She did not tell her colleagues the extent of it. That felt important to her—maintaining the appearance that her relationship with food was a choice, not a concession. She had spent years helping patients navigate illness with honesty and dignity. She could not bring the same honesty to her own. There was something particularly difficult about being a nurse with a condition that her training should have helped her understand. She knew how to explain immune reactivity to a patient. She could not explain why her own reactions kept changing. That gap—between clinical literacy and personal incomprehension—was difficult to reconcile.

Over five years, she tried three separate microbiome protocols. Two gut-directed antimicrobial protocols. An extensive elimination-and-reintroduction diet. A well-designed SIBO treatment protocol. Each had produced temporary improvement. None had held. And with each treatment cycle, the underlying system had become slightly less tolerant, slightly more reactive, slightly more sensitive to inputs that it had previously managed.

"I've watched patients recover from conditions that were far more serious than what I have," she said. "And I keep getting worse. I do everything I know to do and I keep getting worse. What am I missing?"

There was something else in her presentation that none of her previous practitioners had connected to her gut symptoms. Her sleep had been disrupted for several years. She woke consistently between two and four in the morning, could not fall back asleep easily, and felt unrefreshed regardless of how many hours she spent in bed. Her energy followed a strange pattern—lowest in the morning, marginally better in the afternoon, and then a second wind in the evening that made it difficult to wind down before midnight. To most practitioners, this was a separate issue—something to address after the gut was sorted. To me, it was pointing directly at what was holding her gut treatment back.

She was not missing a better treatment. She was missing an understanding of the environment her treatments were entering. And until that environment changed, no treatment aimed at the gut was going to hold.

Three Interdependent Environments

When patients come to me with digestive symptoms, they almost always arrive with a theory. The theory is usually specific, often heavily researched, and built around a single mechanism: candida, SIBO, leaky gut, microbiome imbalance, histamine intolerance, a genetic variant. Some of these theories are correct. Many are partially correct—the finding is real, but it reflects a condition created by a deeper physiologic process rather than the process itself. Treating that condition before the physiology that created it has stabilized is one of the most common causes of treatment failure.

The gut is not a single system. It is three interdependent environments that continuously influence one another, responding to signals from both within the body and from the surrounding environment.

The first environment is the nervous system. The gut has its own nervous system—a network of more than five hundred million neurons embedded in the gut wall, known as the second brain because of the scale and independence of its operations. It is in constant communication with the central nervous system through bidirectional pathways. Far more information travels from the gut to the brain than from the brain to the gut.

When the nervous system is regulated—when the body is operating in states of safety, connection, ease, or pleasure—it sends instructions that support the full machinery of digestion. Blood flow to the gut increases. Motility moves at its natural rhythm. Digestive secretions arrive on schedule. Immune surveillance operates in its default state of educated tolerance.

The microbiome receives the conditions it needs to maintain its diversity and rhythm. This is digestion as it was designed to operate—not because the patient is doing anything special, but because the nervous system is not asking the body to do anything else.

When the nervous system is in sustained threat mode, it sends a different set of instructions. Motility slows or becomes erratic. Blood flow decreases. Immune surveillance in the gut wall increases. The microbiome, which is exquisitely sensitive to changes in the gut environment, shifts its composition in response. This is the body operating under instructions it was never meant to receive continuously. In a substantial proportion of chronic illness cases, gut dysfunction is a consequence of a nervous system that has reorganized the gut's operating environment.

The second environment is the immune-barrier interface. Approximately seventy percent of the body's immune cells reside in the tissues surrounding the gut. This is not incidental. The gut is the largest interface between the outside world and the inside of the body, and the immune system is concentrated there because it must constantly evaluate an enormous volume of incoming information. Food proteins. Microbial fragments. Environmental compounds. Neurotransmitters.

The lining of the gut and the immune tissue beneath it are in continuous negotiation, determining what crosses from the intestine into the body and generating the appropriate response to what does. When the barrier is compromised, the immune system receives inputs it was not designed to process in that form. What follows is not simply a local gut problem. The resulting inflammatory signals can influence physiology throughout the body, affecting tissues and systems far beyond the intestine itself. Immune tolerance breaks down. Foods that were previously tolerated become reactive. The inflammatory tone in the gut wall rises.

The third environment is the microbiome—the ecosystem of bacteria, fungi, and other microorganisms that live in the gut. An adult's gut microbiome contains more individual microorganisms than the human body has cells. These organisms are not bystanders. They help maintain barrier integrity. They regulate immune activity. They produce and influence the production of neurotransmitters, hormones, and chemical messengers.

They generate the short-chain fatty acids that fuel the epithelial cells of the gut wall itself.

The microbiome does not exist independently of the gut's environment. It responds to the conditions created by the nervous system and the immune-barrier interface. Changes in motility, immune activity, diet, sleep, stress, and inflammation all influence which organisms thrive and which decline. The composition of the microbiome therefore reflects the state of the larger system in which it lives.

Because these three environments depend on one another, the order in which they are addressed matters. The treatment sequence follows from this structure.

Each environment shapes the next. The nervous system governs the gut's operating environment. The gut's environment determines what the immune system receives. The immune system's state determines whether the microbiome can stabilize.

The sequence must move from the outside in. Nervous system stability first. Immune regulation second. Barrier restoration and microbiome rebalancing after that. Disrupt any one of these environments and you disturb all three. Address any one of them without addressing the others and the addressed environment will be pulled back toward dysfunction by the unaddressed ones. This is why gut treatment so often fails to hold—not because the wrong thing was targeted, but because the conditions surrounding the target were never changed.

What Was Actually Holding Sophie Back

Sophie had been treating the problem where it appeared: in her gut. The treatments helped, sometimes significantly, but the improvement never lasted. Beneath the symptoms, her immune system remained on alert, repeatedly recreating the same inflammation the protocols were trying to reduce. And that immune vigilance was being sustained by a nervous system that had never received a convincing signal that it was safe to stand down.

For years, Sophie had done everything she believed she needed to do. She learned everything she could. She followed every recommendation. She organized her professional knowledge, her dietary discipline, and her compliance with every protocol around the goal of getting better. The effort had been relentless.

Yet her world continued to grow smaller. The list of foods she trusted kept shrinking. Ordinary meals became negotiations. Travel required planning that often felt more exhausting than staying home. More and more of her life became organized around avoiding the next reaction.

After enough time, the questions began to change. At first, she wondered whether she simply had not found the right treatment. Eventually, she began to wonder whether she had misunderstood the problem itself. The obvious conclusion—that she needed to try something different—was correct. What nobody had offered her was that different might not mean a more intensive treatment. It might mean changing the conditions that allowed the problem to keep returning.

Sophie had reached that point. What nobody had offered her was that the physiology she had been trying to change was responding appropriately to conditions that had never changed.

But there was a second layer to her stall—one that her sleep pattern had been trying to communicate for years, and that required understanding something about the microbiome that is often overlooked when gut problems are viewed only through the lenses of digestion, inflammation, and microbial composition.

The microbiome has a rhythm.

This is not a metaphor. Its influence depends not only on which organisms are present, but also on how their activity is organized over time. When that organization is lost, the consequences reach beyond the gut.

The Microbiome's Reach Beyond the Gut

The microbiome does not just respond to the body's clock. It helps regulate it.

Many features of the gut microbiome follow daily rhythms. Microbial populations change in abundance and activity across the day, and the metabolites they produce help coordinate the timing of immune activity, metabolism, and other physiologic processes. When this microbial rhythmicity remains intact, it reinforces the body's broader daily organization and supports the overnight physiology involved in barrier maintenance, immune regulation, and inflammatory resolution.

Dysbiosis and circadian disruption can flatten or disorganize those microbial oscillations. The timing signals become less consistent. Overnight repair and immune regulation may become less complete. Inflammation that should have resolved can carry forward into the next day, leaving the immune system more activated than it should be.

Sophie's sleep pattern suggested that her gut dysfunction and circadian disruption might not have been separate problems. Her previous treatments had addressed bacterial overgrowth and barrier permeability—both real problems. What they had not addressed were the timing and environmental conditions helping organize microbial behavior.

Her gut dysfunction could disrupt circadian organization. Poor sleep and circadian disruption could, in turn, interfere with immune regulation and make the gut environment harder to stabilize. The microbiome was not the sole cause of all three problems, but it participated in the loop connecting them.

When circadian function fails to improve despite appropriate sleep and light-based interventions, the problem may not begin with sleep itself. An unresolved gut-immune disturbance may still be preventing the circadian system from stabilizing.

Change the conditions, and the biology changes with them. Leave the conditions unchanged, and the biology has little reason to do anything different.

Why the Loop Keeps Running

Gut inflammation often regenerates even after the dietary triggers are removed, the barrier is supported, and the antimicrobial protocol has been completed correctly.

The inflammatory signaling is not being regenerated by food or bacteria alone. The overnight repair window is where the immune system would normally complete its resolution of the day's inflammation. That process depends, in part, on the microbiome's rhythmic organization. When that rhythm is disrupted, the overnight repair window can no longer complete the work it was designed to do. Inflammation that should have cleared by morning persists into the next day. And the food reactions the patient was hoping would improve after another week of careful eating remain exactly as they were.

Consider what this feels like from inside the experience. The patient has been following their protocol carefully. They have removed the trigger foods. They have taken probiotics and gut-support supplements. They have completed the antimicrobial protocol. They have been patient. And Monday morning arrives with the same bloating, the same brain fog, the same urgency that was there six weeks ago.

The protocol has not failed them. The overnight repair cycle has.

Stabilize Before You Escalate

Once the regulation gate has been passed—once the nervous system has achieved sufficient stability—the immune system begins to receive different instructions. The inflammatory tone begins to subside. The gut immune tissue begins to shift from reactive surveillance toward education and tolerance. And the barrier begins to have the physiologic space to repair.

This transition follows its own sequence. The microbiome's rhythmicity must be restored alongside its composition. Almost all gut treatment protocols address composition without addressing rhythmicity. They reintroduce probiotics and prebiotics to support their growth, but the environment those bacteria enter—dysregulated in its timing, deprived of the circadian cues that organize microbial behavior—cannot support the new composition. The new composition does not stabilize. Improvement does not hold.

The opposite mistake is just as common. Antimicrobial protocols reduce bacterial abundance and diversity along with the organisms they are intended to remove. When that loss occurs in a microbiome whose rhythmic organization is already disrupted, recovery becomes even more difficult. The ecosystem has now lost both its composition and the rhythmic organization that helps keep it stable. Rebuilding from this state requires restoring both.

This is the pattern Sophie had lived through five times. Each time a protocol produced temporary improvement, the conclusion was that the protocol had not been sufficient. The dosing was increased. The antimicrobial was changed. The elimination diet was extended. The intervention was escalated rather than questioned. And each escalation produced a smaller improvement than the last, because each escalation added more treatment load to a system that was already spending more resources adapting to the treatment than it was gaining from it.

When something is not improving at this layer, the instinct is almost always to escalate—to add a stronger antimicrobial, a more intensive protocol, a more restrictive diet. That instinct is almost always wrong. The correct question is not what more can be done. It is whether the foundation beneath the gut dysfunction is stable enough to support what is already being attempted. Stabilize before you escalate. The goal is not to do less. The goal is to stop asking the next layer to compensate for a layer that has not yet stabilized.

You cannot permanently fix the microbiome while its supporting systems remain dysregulated.

Every unsuccessful intervention creates pressure to do more. More supplements. More restrictions. More testing. More treatment. But biology is not impressed by effort. Escalation is seductive because it feels active. Stabilization can feel like very little is happening. Yet stabilization is frequently the intervention that determines whether anything else will work.

This is why patients often feel genuinely better for weeks or even months before gradually finding themselves back where they started. The treatment changed the microbiome. But the conditions governing microbial behavior—its timing, its rhythm, its nervous system tone, its overnight repair capacity—never changed. The new microbial composition could not sustain itself inside the same conditions that had produced the original dysbiosis. The patient concludes they must have chosen the wrong protocol, have resistant bacteria, or still have hidden food triggers. In most cases, what they have is an environment that was never addressed. The microbiome responds to its environment. When that environment becomes stable, it can return to equilibrium with the other systems of the body.

Those conditions are not simply the chemical composition of the gut. They include its timing, its rhythm, and the circadian organization of the gut ecosystem. Restore the rhythm alongside the composition, and the microbiome can hold what you give it.

The Food Reaction Paradox

One observation changes how patients understand food reactions—and, just as importantly, how they live around them.

In a system with compromised barrier function and chronic immune activation, food reactions do not reflect which foods are problematic and which are safe. They reflect the current state of the immune system's tolerance. That tolerance changes as the underlying conditions change.

This explains why the list of tolerated foods often keeps shrinking, even in patients who are doing everything their practitioners recommend. The immune system is not malfunctioning when it reacts to a new food.

It is functioning exactly as a compromised immune system should—with less tolerance, more reactivity, and less margin for variation. The barrier is more permeable than it should be. Materials that should remain inside the gut begin crossing into the tissue, where the immune system must decide how to respond. The tissue operates in a state of heightened surveillance that is appropriate to the inputs it is receiving. The problem is not the immune response. The problem is the conditions producing the inputs that require that response.

This distinction changes the goal of treatment. If the immune system is viewed as the problem, the goal becomes suppressing the response. If the immune system is viewed as responding appropriately, the goal shifts: change what it is responding to. The conditions producing those inputs must change. The barrier must become more selective. The inflammatory signaling must decrease. The nervous system must begin signaling safety instead of sustained threat. When those conditions change, the immune response usually changes with them—not because the immune system was forced to behave differently, but because the information it was responding to has changed.

The food reactions are real. They are not imagined. The immune system is genuinely responding to materials crossing a compromised barrier in a form that triggers reactivity. The discomfort, the inflammation, the brain fog—these are real physiologic events.

And the list of reactive foods is not fixed. Sophie's list had been shrinking for three years because her immune tolerance had been progressively declining as the underlying conditions driving it remained unaddressed.

This is also why the search for the one bad food rarely produces an answer. The patient who has been told their reactions are real and physiologic often concludes that the next step is to identify exactly which foods are responsible. But in a system whose tolerance is narrowing, the variable that is changing is not which foods are reactive. It is the immune system's threshold for reactivity. As that threshold changes, the list grows. The foods are not the moving part.

A shrinking food list gradually becomes a life in contraction. The food planning begins to consume a significant portion of daily cognitive energy. Every invitation involving a meal becomes a calculation: what will be available, what the risk is, whether the social cost of explaining is higher than the cost of declining. Restaurants are vetted in advance. Safe foods are carried in bags and purses as insurance. Eating away from home becomes something to be managed rather than enjoyed, and eventually something to be avoided. Social life narrows along the same radius as the diet. What began as a medical strategy gradually becomes a way of life. The restrictions stop feeling temporary and start feeling permanent. The person living inside them knows they are not getting better. They are simply working harder to avoid getting worse.

Avoidance manages symptoms. It does not restore tolerance. The immune system builds and maintains tolerance to familiar food proteins through repeated, consistent exposure over time. When those proteins are eliminated, the immune system has no opportunity to recalibrate its response. In a system whose tolerance is still narrowing, avoidance alone means the list of safe foods will continue to shrink regardless of how carefully the elimination is maintained.

The most effective treatment for food reactivity is almost never directly targeted at the foods themselves. It is targeted at the gut barrier, the microbiome's rhythmicity, and above all, the nervous system and immune environment driving the entire cascade. When those layers stabilize, the food reactions resolve as a downstream consequence.

Foundation Work You Can Do Now

The practice for this chapter requires two kinds of consistency, applied simultaneously. Neither requires identifying and eliminating specific reactive foods beyond any foods you already know you are truly allergic to. If you have a diagnosed food allergy or have experienced a severe allergic reaction, continue avoiding those foods. Both require only that the gut receive the same signals, at the same times, in the same sequence, for long enough that the environment begins to organize around them.

Between meals, the gut runs a housekeeping program called the migrating motor complex—a coordinated wave of muscular contractions that sweeps residual food particles, bacteria, and cellular debris from the small intestine toward the colon. It runs every ninety minutes to two hours during fasted states, and it only runs when the gut is not actively digesting. In a system that grazes constantly, the migrating motor complex rarely completes its cycle. Material that should have been cleared remains in the small intestine. Transit slows. Constipation becomes more likely. Bacterial overgrowth can accumulate. The barrier becomes more permeable. Immune activation rises.

Consistent meal timing—eating at predictable intervals with genuine fasted periods between complete meals—allows the migrating motor complex to run its full cycle. The practical application: eat at consistent times each day, and allow at least four hours between complete eating episodes. If you are currently grazing throughout the day, begin by consolidating into three consistent meal times.

Meal timing is not just a gut intervention. It is an act of environmental organization. Regular meals at consistent times tell the entire gut ecosystem—and the circadian system above it—that the day is predictable, that the environment can be trusted, that it is safe to run the repair cycles that nighttime requires. The body predicts safety partly through rhythm. This is the same principle that governs the nervous system's response to routine, discussed in Chapter 5. Predictability reduces vigilance. Reduced vigilance permits restoration. The gut responds to that principle the same way the nervous system does.

The second consistency is dietary stability during the stabilization period.

Eat the same core foods for two to four weeks. Not the same meals, but the same ingredients, prepared in ways you tolerate well, without introducing new foods during this period of stabilization. When inputs vary constantly, the immune system cannot build reliable predictions about what it should tolerate. Consistent inputs give the immune system the stability it needs to begin recalibrating.

When the same foods arrive at roughly the same times each day, the microbiome's activity becomes more predictable. That predictability strengthens everything downstream of it—the body's daily rhythms, the overnight repair cycle, and the immune system's ability to complete its work before morning.

These two practices are not a permanent prescription. They are a phase of stabilization. The goal is not to eat the same thing forever. The goal is to create the conditions under which the immune system can begin restoring its tolerance; the microbiome can restore its rhythmicity; and the circadian clock can once again receive the signals it needs to generate the overnight repair on which everything else depends.

After establishing the nervous system foundation described in the previous chapter, Sophie began with these two practices. Eight weeks later, for the first time in three years, her list of reactive foods had stopped growing. Ten weeks after that, something she had not expected: her sleep began to improve. Not dramatically—but enough that she knew something was changing. She was waking less frequently. The two-to-four AM window that had disrupted her sleep for years began to shorten. Her morning energy began arriving slightly earlier.

Nothing had been done directly for her sleep. What had changed were the upstream conditions preventing it from improving. The microbiome's metabolic rhythm was beginning to recover. The body's own sleep chemistry was beginning to recover with it. And sleep—not as a target, but as a consequence—was beginning to follow.

She described the change as a reduction of effort. The meals were still simple. The routine was still deliberate. The constant vigilance—the background hum of monitoring and managing and preparing for the next reaction—had begun to quiet.

She stopped vetting restaurants before she went somewhere. Not completely—not yet. But one Thursday she accepted a lunch invitation from a colleague without looking up the restaurant first. She brought nothing as backup. She ate what was available and came back to her shift without it becoming the subject of that afternoon's calculation. It was an ordinary lunch. That was the point.

"I thought the sleep and the gut were two separate problems," she told me. "I had no idea they were the same environment."

They were not the same problem. But they shared the same upstream driver. And that is the distinction that changes everything about how recovery is approached.

Sophie's recovery did not happen because her immune system was treated. It happened because the conditions surrounding her immune system began to organize.

# # #

CHAPTER SEVEN

The Clock Your Body Runs On

"The problem is rarely that the patient is not sleeping.
The problem is that the body is not entering restorative sleep.
Those are not the same thing.
And treating one as though it were the other
is why sleep treatment so often fails."
—Marcus Ettinger, DC

Thomas

His name is Thomas. He was sixty-one years old, a recently retired chemistry professor who had taught at the same university for twenty-four years. He had not planned to retire. Not yet. He had always planned to teach as long as the university would have him.

Chemistry had been, for as long as he could remember, the way he made sense of the world. He liked equations because they balanced. He liked experiments because the answer was either there or it wasn't, and you could find out which by being careful. Thomas had built a career around making chemistry understandable to undergraduates who arrived in his classroom convinced it was going to be the hardest course of their semester and left, in a meaningful percentage of cases, having enjoyed it. He was good at it. He had been the kind of professor whose former students emailed him fifteen years later to tell him what they were doing.

His wife Rebecca—Becca, to him, since the first month they had been dating—had been part of this life for twenty-four years. They had a chemistry of their own, the kind that made other people comment, and most of their adult social life had been organized around two pursuits in which Thomas had excelled and in which Becca had been the indispensable partner. He brewed beer, seriously and competitively, in a club that ran tastings and regional competitions. He smoked meat—low-and-slow, Texas-style, on an offset Yoder that took eighteen hours to do brisket properly—and entered BBQ contests three or four times a year. He won regularly at both. The reason he won—as he stated proudly to his friends, more than once—was that brewing and smoking were eight parts chemistry and two parts passion.

The trouble had started so gradually that for the first two years he attributed it to age. He was tired in the morning. Then he was tired all day. His memory, which had been the thing he was known for in his department—the iron trap, his graduate students used to call it—began to slip in ways that he could initially talk himself out of noticing. He would lose the thread of an equation he had carried in his head for thirty years. He would walk into the lab and, for a moment that felt longer than it was, forget why he had gone there. He started relying on notes for simple tasks that had always lived easily in his head.

He compensated, the way competent people compensate. He relied on his assistant more than he had ever relied on anyone in his career. He double-checked work he would not have double-checked before. He scheduled the cognitive work that mattered most for the hours of the day when he felt closest to himself, which was usually the late afternoon, and arranged the rest of his day around protecting that window. From the outside, he was a professor in his late fifties, slightly more cautious than he used to be. From the inside, he was a man who was no longer sure he could be trusted with the work he spent his life doing.

He resigned the year he turned fifty-nine. The official reason was retirement. The actual reason was that there had been an afternoon in the lab when he could not remember, with certainty, whether he had calibrated an instrument that morning. He had calibrated it. He found the log entry.

But the not-knowing had frightened him in a way that he could not unfeel. He submitted his resignation letter four weeks later. He told Becca it had been a long time coming. He told his department chair the same. He did not tell either of them about the calibration.

What followed was harder to describe than the resignation. The brewing slowed first. A new batch of beer required a week of preparation, careful temperature control, and the kind of patient attention to fermentation that did not forgive a missed step. He could still do it. But the day after, he would be unable to do anything else, and the day after that, the same. He stopped entering competitions because the timing of the contests required him to commit, weeks ahead, to being functional on a particular weekend. He could not predict whether he would be. So he stopped agreeing.

The BBQ followed. An eighteen-hour cook required him to wake every two hours through the night to manage the temperature of the smoker. Thomas had loved this once—the dark hours alone with the smell of post-oak and the slow chemistry of collagen breaking down into something his friends would still be talking about a year later. After he turned sixty, he did one competition and was useless for three days afterward. He did not enter another. The Yoder sat covered on the patio. He used it occasionally, for the family, for shorter cooks that did not punish him.

He and Becca had been the social anchor of a brewing club and a BBQ circuit for nearly twenty years. The friendships were real. The competitions had been the structure that brought everyone together. When Thomas stopped competing, the invitations slowed. He had not been pushed out. He simply stopped saying yes to things he was no longer sure he could do, and after enough months of that, people stopped asking. Becca had watched this happen without entirely understanding it. She knew he was tired. She did not know how carefully he had begun to count what he could spend.

"My wife says I sleep fine," he told me. "She's right. I sleep fine. I just don't feel like it."

He fell asleep without difficulty. He stayed asleep. He slept between seven and eight hours on most nights. He had a sleep tracker that had been confirming this for three years. The data was consistent. The data made no sense to him, because he woke every morning feeling exactly as unrestored as he had felt going to bed, and no adjustment to the inputs he could measure had changed that.

Thomas had tried what a meticulous person tries. Fixed wake time. Bedroom temperature calibrated to sixty-eight degrees. No screens after nine. Blackout curtains. A magnesium supplement at eight-thirty. A wind-down routine that he maintained for two years without deviation. Caffeine had been removed for six weeks. He experimented with sleep restriction therapy, which had actually made things worse, and with extended sleep opportunities, which had produced no noticeable improvement. He varied his exercise timing, his meal timing, and his light exposure. The variables accumulated. No pattern emerged that responded to the adjustments.

The problem was not that Thomas had never encountered the right pieces. He had. The problem was that he was treating them as isolated sleep interventions rather than as signals to a circadian system that had lost its timing. Many of the individual practices were familiar. The sequence they belonged to was not.

"I keep thinking I'll figure it out," he said. "I know how to figure things out. I've been figuring things out my whole life. And I can't figure this out."

What he was describing, when I asked him to walk me through a full day rather than just his nights, filled in a picture the sleep tracker had not captured. He had no functional energy in the morning and required two cups of coffee before he felt capable of sustained thought. By mid-afternoon the first round of caffeine was wearing off, and he managed the crash with a third cup. He had a reliable energy window in the late afternoon—usually between four and six—when he felt closest to himself. He could not fall asleep before midnight despite being genuinely tired by nine, because tired was not the same as sleepy. Sleepy did not arrive on schedule. He woke at six, reliably, not from an alarm but from some internal signal, feeling exactly as unrestored as when he had gone to bed.

The larger pattern took longer to surface, and he did not state it directly. He stated it through what he had stopped doing. The brewing competitions. The BBQ circuit. The summer trip he and Becca used to take with another couple. The weekend visits to their daughter's family three hours north—the ones that involved staying overnight, because he could not predict how he would feel the next morning. Thomas had three grandchildren under the age of seven. He saw them often, but had not slept in the same house with them in more than two years.

What he was describing was a circadian system running flat and late, an internal clock that was generating the wrong signal at the wrong time and had been doing so for long enough that he had stopped trying to plan around it. He had not lost his energy. He had lost his ability to predict it. And a life, it turns out, is not built on energy. A life is built on the assumption that next Saturday you will still be the person you are today. When that assumption begins to fail enough, you do what Thomas had done. You make the life smaller. You decline what you cannot guarantee. You become, by careful subtraction, someone you would not have recognized ten years earlier.

Thomas had been trying to fix his sleep. The clock that determined whether sleep restored him—the clock that had been running flat and late for longer than he had been measuring—could not be fixed by any of the inputs he tried. It had to be given the conditions to recover.

What the Clock Actually Does

Sleep is not a thing that happens to you at night. It is the culmination of a process that begins the moment you wake up in the morning. The quality of the sleep you get tonight is determined, in large part, by how well every system in your body has maintained its timing across the preceding sixteen hours.

Sleep is governed by two cooperating forces. One is the pressure to sleep, which builds the longer you remain awake. The other is the circadian signal that determines when the brain is prepared to act on that pressure. You can therefore be profoundly tired without being physiologically ready for sleep, or sleep for many hours without moving through the stages and cycles that make those hours restorative.

The circadian system provides the timing half of this relationship. It is the biological clock that governs the daily rhythm of virtually every physiologic function in your body. Cortisol. Melatonin. Body temperature. Immune activity. Digestive function. Cell repair. All of these cycle in a predictable daily pattern, orchestrated by a master clock in the brain that is synchronized by light—specifically, the daily cycle of sunlight and darkness—and communicates precise timing signals to every organ through a cascade of hormonal and neural messages.

When this clock is running well, sleep is not a problem. The body knows when to be alert and when to rest. It makes the transitions between those states naturally. Morning arrives with genuine energy. Evening arrives with genuine tiredness. The night provides the repair that the day requires.

The brain's master clock coordinates not just the brain's own activities but every peripheral clock in the body—the liver, the gut, the immune system, the muscles, and even the daily rhythms of the gut microbiome, whose activity changes across the day in response to the body's timing signals. Each organ runs its own local timing program, performing its specific maintenance and repair work during the windows the central clock designates for it. When those windows are correctly timed and the signals are strong, the body's repair systems work in coordinated sequence. When the clock's signal is weak or delayed, the peripheral clocks drift. The liver is trying to run in night-mode while the gut is still in day-mode. The immune system is activating when it should be repairing. The muscles are receiving recovery signals after the window for efficient repair has already begun to close.

This is what was happening to Thomas. Not a single system failing. His entire timing architecture was operating too quietly and too late, so the repair his sleep hours were supposed to enable was chronically incomplete.

Two Ways the Clock Fails

In clinical practice, circadian dysfunction in chronic illness does not always present the same way. Two common patterns stand out from the rest. Understanding which pattern predominates helps explain why patients with similar complaints can respond differently to the same intervention.

The first pattern is a clock that speaks too quietly—what I call amplitude failure. The circadian clock is still running, but its signal has become too weak. The distinction between day and night is still present, but the contrast has faded. Morning activation is present but muted. Evening sleepiness still arrives, but with less strength than it should.

Everything is present, but at half volume. Energy remains relatively flat across the day instead of rising strongly in the morning and falling naturally at night. Sleep occurs, but it is often shallow and fails to become deeply restorative. Patients commonly describe feeling "never fully awake during the day and never fully asleep at night"—and that description is physiologically accurate.

The second pattern is a body that no longer responds reliably to the clock—what I call output signaling failure. Here the circadian clock still keeps accurate time. Morning arrives on schedule. The body does not. The day begins before the body is ready for it. Hours may pass before energy, alertness, digestion, and mental clarity begin to follow. The morning cortisol rise may be delayed or blunted. The body is no longer preparing for the day before the day begins. Instead, it is reacting to the day after it has already started. Eventually, many patients stop planning mornings because they can no longer rely on them.

The initial focus differs depending on which pattern predominates. Amplitude failure responds to stronger environmental cues—more consistent morning light, more deliberate evening light reduction, tighter meal timing. Output signaling failure responds to precision and structure—exact wake time consistency, morning protein at a consistent time, and structured morning activation before asking anything of the body. Treating an output signaling failure as though it were an amplitude problem often prolongs the stall because the body has not yet relearned how to respond reliably to circadian cues. Treating an amplitude failure as an output problem usually still produces improvement, but often more slowly and with unnecessary complexity because the additional precision is not yet required.

The distinction matters because it changes the emphasis and precision of treatment, not the foundational principles of recovery.

Not all unrefreshing sleep stems from circadian dysfunction. Sleep apnea, primary insomnia, medication effects, alcohol before bed, and other sleep disorders or physiologic disruptions can all produce the same exhausted-but-not-rested feeling, and each requires its own careful assessment. Amplitude failure and output signaling failure are clinical patterns I use to interpret where circadian restoration may be stalling. They are not formal sleep-disorder diagnoses and do not replace a thorough clinical evaluation of sleep in its full complexity.

The Tired But Wired Pattern

Thomas was living in one common pattern of circadian dysfunction—a clock running too quietly and too late. Another common presentation cannot be explained by circadian timing alone. It is the "tired but wired" pattern—the state of being genuinely fatigued while simultaneously unable to disengage from the environment. The body wants to rest. The brain will not allow it. Evening arrives with exhaustion but not with the quieting of environmental monitoring that is supposed to accompany it.

You are lying in bed, genuinely tired, and you can hear every sound in the house—the refrigerator cycling, a car passing outside, the ambient settling of the building. You are aware of them with a clarity that belongs to daytime.

Over time, many people begin to dread bedtime because they already know the sequence that is about to unfold. They will be tired. They will be ready for sleep. And then they will spend the next hour negotiating with a brain that refuses to leave the day behind. The bed becomes associated with effort rather than rest.

Your thoughts do not slow. They maintain the same looping, associative quality they have during the day, moving from one unresolved item to the next instead of gradually softening as sleep approaches. The awareness never dims. You cannot "fall away" from the world, which is exactly what sleep requires you to do. You are not anxious, necessarily. You are simply present—physiologically alert—in a body exhausted by remaining engaged but still waiting for the signal that it can stop.

Sleep begins when the brain stops reacting to the environment—not just when the body becomes tired. This distinction is clinically critical. A patient who is tired but cannot sleep is not simply lacking the drive to sleep. What they are experiencing is a failure of sensory disengagement. The brain is still tracking, evaluating, and responding to environmental input when it should be withdrawing from it.

Melatonin is one of the principal chemical signals behind the evening dimmer switch—not primarily a sedative, but a message that night has arrived and the brain's responsiveness to the environment should begin to decrease. When that signal rises on schedule, it helps the brain disengage from the day. When it is delayed or blunted, environmental surveillance can continue into the night, leaving the person exhausted but unable to cross the threshold into sleep.

Sleep does not begin when the body becomes tired enough. It begins when the brain's sleep-promoting systems are able to quiet the networks that keep it engaged with the world. Circadian timing helps determine when that transition can occur. It cannot be forced. It can only be supported by restoring the conditions that allow the clock and the sleep system to work together.

When Viral Illness Disrupts the Clock

There is a specific cause of the amplitude failure pattern that deserves separate attention—one that follows acute viral illness and is often missed because patients and clinicians both assume that recovery from the infection means recovery of the whole person. The infection ends. Energy is supposed to return. When it does not, the patient is often told that the illness is "in the past" and that the lingering fatigue must come from something else.

Sometimes the illness has ended, but its effects on the systems responsible for recovery have not. The inflammation that the immune system produces during a serious viral illness does not always end when the virus does. Sometimes it lingers in the parts of the brain that regulate the daily clock—the same structures that help determine when cortisol should rise in the morning and when melatonin should rise in the evening.

When the inflammation persists, the clock no longer keeps time the way it should. Patients describe waking each morning feeling as though their bodies are still asleep long after they are awake. They describe energy that arrives in the late afternoon when they need it in the morning. They describe sleep that, even after eight hours, never seems to deliver them back to themselves.

This pattern has long been recognized following Epstein-Barr virus, influenza, and many other viral illnesses. The COVID-19 pandemic simply made it visible on a scale that was difficult to ignore.

This is the same amplitude failure pattern Thomas had lived in, triggered by a different cause. The intervention sequence is the same. The timeline for restoration is often longer because the inflammation that drives the disruption can take months to fully resolve even after the infection itself is gone.

What Phase 3 Is Actually Doing for Phase 4

Patients often report something surprising as they move into Phase 4: their sleep keeps improving even though they are no longer focused on it. The deeper their recovery becomes, the deeper their sleep becomes with it.

This is not a coincidence. The circadian clock and the mitochondria—the structures inside cells that generate energy—operate through a two-way relationship. The clock influences mitochondrial function. Mitochondrial function influences the clock.

Most people intuitively understand the first half of this relationship. The circadian clock tells the mitochondria when to produce more energy, when to perform maintenance, and when to shift into conservation mode. When that timing is consistent, energy becomes more predictable. Patients notice fewer unexpected crashes, steadier mental clarity, quicker recovery after physical or mental effort, and a growing confidence that tomorrow will be a better day.

The other half of the relationship is what changes how you understand Phase 3 in the context of the whole hierarchy. As mitochondrial efficiency improves—through the restoration of consistent, deep sleep and the recovery it enables—the circadian signal strengthens in return. Patients notice this before they understand it. The clock's timing becomes more precise. The amplitude of the signal increases. The day-night contrast improves. The loop reinforces itself.

The clinical consequence is something I observe regularly: as Phase 4 progresses, patients often report that their sleep deepens further without any additional sleep intervention. This is the feedback loop becoming visible. Phase 4 is strengthening Phase 3—not because anything new was done for sleep, but because the hierarchy, respected in the right sequence, began to reinforce itself.

The loop also runs in the other direction. Phase 4 regression—through over-demand or premature escalation—can destabilize Phase 3 gains. This often happens when patients begin asking more of their bodies before their recovery capacity has fully returned. Exercise intensifies too quickly. Long workdays resume. Travel, fasting, or additional therapies are introduced faster than the system can organize around them. Sleep quality becomes lighter and less restorative. Morning energy begins to fade. Recovery after physical or mental effort takes longer again.

Because declining energy is usually the first change patients notice, both the patient and practitioner often conclude that the problem has begun in the energy layer. But symptoms often appear where the hierarchy finally fails, not where the disruption first began. The circadian layer had already begun to lose its stability. The decline in energy simply exposed the earlier problem.

This is why Phase 3 is not merely preparation for Phase 4. It is the foundation that Phase 4 depends on throughout its entire course.

What Restores the Clock

What restores the clock is not primarily a medication or supplement. It is a set of environmental timing cues. Chronobiologists call these cues zeitgebers—literally "time-givers"—because they continually synchronize the body's internal clock to the external world. If timing has been lost, timing must be restored.

No single timing cue restores the clock by itself. Each strengthens the others. Together they provide the repeated daily information the circadian system uses to recover its rhythm. The most powerful of these signals is light. Morning light exposure—particularly outdoor light in the first thirty minutes after waking—gives the master clock the timing reference it needs to anchor the day's rhythm. Outdoor light intensity, even on overcast days, is dramatically higher than that of typical indoor lighting. The eye registers the difference even when conscious awareness does not. Patients who begin stepping outside within the first half hour of waking often report that mornings gradually begin to feel different—that their day starts when they do rather than several hours later.

Evening light reduction matters just as much. Dimming indoor lights after sunset, reducing screen exposure, avoiding the blue-spectrum light that mimics daylight—these are not relaxation strategies. They are signals to the body that the day is ending. For most people living in the modern world, the evening melatonin signal is chronically delayed simply by the light environment they live in, even in the absence of any underlying illness. The bedroom that stays bright until midnight is not just disruptive. It is, to the circadian system, indistinguishable from afternoon.

The next most powerful timing cue is the first meal of the day. Consistently timing that meal helps synchronize the liver, gut, muscle, and other peripheral clocks with the rest of the circadian system. In my clinical experience, a protein-containing breakfast within the first hour after waking often provides the clearest metabolic signal. Without consistent meal timing, these peripheral clocks receive a weaker timing signal, and the rest of the day's rhythm begins to drift. This is the same meal-timing principle discussed in Chapter 6 from the perspective of gut health. Here it appears again from the perspective of circadian biology. The same behavior addresses both simultaneously.

Consistent physical activity performed at a consistent time provides another important circadian signal. In Phase 3, exercise is not yet a training stimulus. It is a timing cue. Whenever possible, perform it during daylight hours, when the exercise reinforces rather than competes with the body's natural light signals. The question is not how hard to exercise. It is when, and whether the consistency improves the rhythm.

The foundational signal that ties all the others together is waking at the same time each day. Doing this every morning, regardless of how well you slept, provides the master clock with one of its most reliable anchoring cues. The body cannot keep accurate time on its own. It has to be calibrated by its environment. Wake time is, for the circadian system, what the breathing practice is for the nervous system: a simple daily practice that allows every other circadian signal to work more effectively.

Foundation Work You Can Do Now

The practical work of this chapter builds directly on what you have already established. The consistent wake time from Chapter 2, the consistent meal timing from Chapter 6, the evening wind-down anchor from Chapter 5—these are all circadian interventions. They work because they are timing cues the clock can use to anchor its rhythm.

What this chapter adds is the light dimension.

Within the first thirty minutes of waking, get bright light. Outdoor light is preferred. Go outside not to exercise, not to accomplish anything, not to check your phone, but simply to be in the morning light. Ten to twenty minutes may be sufficient on a clear day. On an overcast day, go anyway and stay longer. If outdoor light is unavailable, use a ten-thousand-lux light therapy box during the same morning window for approximately twenty to thirty minutes. It is a reasonable alternative, but it does not fully reproduce the intensity, spectrum, and natural variability of outdoor light. For readers living in regions where daylight becomes unusually prolonged or limited during parts of the year, the principle does not change: the clock still needs a reliable signal that morning has begun.

Do not wear sunglasses during this practice. The intensity of the light environment, experienced by unshielded eyes, is what provides the cue.

Beginning sixty to ninety minutes before your target sleep time, reduce indoor light intensity meaningfully. Dimmer switches, floor lamps instead of overhead lights, or simply turning off unnecessary lights will accomplish this. If you use screens in the evening, reduce their brightness, switch to the warmest available color temperature, and try to stop using them at least thirty minutes before sleep.

If you find yourself consistently alert and environmentally responsive at night despite being genuinely tired, add ten minutes of slow rhythmic breathing—four to six seconds in, six seconds out—approximately forty-five minutes before your target sleep time. The breathing practice from Chapter 3, applied here at a specific time with a specific goal: to begin the autonomic downshift. The breathing lowers the body's activation. The melatonin signal—arriving on a better-functioning clock—can then finish the work of letting go of the day.

Thomas began the protocol the way he began everything: methodically, carefully, with notes. He went outside in the first thirty minutes after waking. He turned the lights down ninety minutes before bed. He kept the wake time consistent. He added the slow rhythmic breathing some evenings when the tired-but-wired pattern showed up.

For the first month, nothing he could measure changed. He told me he had expected this. He told me, more honestly, that he had also expected to feel discouraged, and was working not to.

Around the seventh or eighth week, Becca noticed something before he did. She said that he had been getting up before her three or four mornings in a row, and that he was no longer sitting on the edge of the bed for several minutes while he assembled himself. She mentioned it casually. He had not been aware of it. At twelve weeks, the change he could measure was small but no longer ambiguous. He was waking earlier, before the alarm, on most mornings. The morning coffee was still there but he was not waiting for it before he could think. The afternoon crash was no longer reliable enough to plan around. He had stopped tracking, somewhere around week ten, because tracking had stopped being interesting.

Something else changed as well. He was losing the thread less often. The small lapses that once made him question himself—walking into a room and forgetting why he had gone there, reaching for notes he had never needed before—were becoming less common. He gave it little thought until he suddenly realized he had stopped monitoring his own mind so closely.

What was happening underneath what he could feel was that a clock which had been running flat and late for more than a decade was beginning, slowly, to recover its amplitude and timing. The morning light was anchoring the master clock to the actual day. The evening darkness was permitting melatonin to arrive on schedule. The consistent wake time was giving the system a reference point to stabilize around. None of these interventions were doing the recovery. They were giving the clock the conditions it needed to do what it had always been designed to do.

The realization did not come one morning. It came on an ordinary Tuesday afternoon. He and Becca had been invited to a regional BBQ competition seven weeks out—an event he had been part of for fifteen years before stopping. The invitation had come by text from an old friend who said the team needed another set of hands and an honest tongue. Becca read the text aloud over lunch. Thomas said yes before he had thought about whether he should. He never stopped to calculate the true cost of that eighteen-hour cook. He never paused to wonder whether he would still be functional the next morning, or the day after that. For the first time in four years, he simply said yes.

An hour later, he recognized what he had just done.

He told me this with the quietness of someone describing something he did not yet fully understand.

"I just said yes. I haven't said yes to something like that in a long time."

He was sixty-two when he and Becca drove to that competition. Their team placed second in pork shoulder. He was tired the day after. He was not destroyed. He slept that night and the next. The next morning he woke and stayed in bed for a few minutes in a way he had not been able to in years—not because he had to gather himself, but because he wanted to lie there a little longer.

Three weeks later, he and Becca drove up to their daughter's house and stayed two nights. He woke both mornings in the unfamiliar guest room and got up to make coffee in his daughter's kitchen. There was no negotiation. He played with the grandchildren before lunch in the backyard and was tired afterward, but not in the way he had been tired for the past several years. He was tired the way someone who had spent a morning chasing small children should be tired.

"I didn't know that was supposed to happen," he told me. "I thought morning tiredness was just how I was."

It was not how he was. It was how his clock had been running. And clocks, given the right conditions for long enough, can recover what they were designed to do.

Trust in tomorrow is one thing. Trust that effort will be followed by recovery is the next.

CHAPTER EIGHT

Earning Energy

"The body does not withhold energy because it has forgotten how to produce it. It withholds energy because the conditions for recovery have not been met. Earning energy is not about pushing harder. It is about demonstrating, repeatedly, that the demand can be met and recovered from."
—Marcus Ettinger, DC

David

His name is David. He was fifty-one years old, and he had been running four or five mornings a week for most of his adult life. Not competitively—he had never been particularly interested in race times or performance metrics. He ran because it worked. It was how he processed stress. After a difficult day, a difficult week, a difficult year, the run returned him to himself. It had been doing that reliably for more than two decades.

Running had carried him through his father's illness. Through a professional setback that had cost him two years of work. Through the year both his children left for college within the same twelve months, and the house went quiet in a way he had not anticipated. He had never thought of himself as someone who depended on exercise for his emotional equilibrium. He had simply noticed, across twenty years, that the difficult things in his life were more manageable after a run. And when they were not, he ran again.

The ceiling appeared gradually, over about eighteen months, and at first he could not tell whether it was real.

The runs felt the same during the sessions themselves—the effort was familiar, the pace was consistent, nothing was dramatically different in the moment. But something was different afterward. He was finishing runs and feeling more depleted than the distance should have produced. He was sleeping eight hours and was still waking up tired. He was having productive days—genuinely productive, by any reasonable measure—and paying for them over the following forty-eight hours with a fatigue that made those days feel borrowed.

The pattern that disturbed him most was the one he called the good week problem. He would have four or five days of feeling genuinely functional—training well, working well, sleeping adequately—and then something would shift. Not dramatically. Not a crash he could point to as a cause. Just a week that suddenly required more management than the previous one had. He began keeping notes, looking for the variable. He could not find it.

"I feel fine during the run," he told me. "And then the run costs me two days. And I don't understand why a run that felt normal is costing me two days."

He had started adjusting. He reduced his weekly mileage. He added recovery days. He changed his sleep schedule, updated his diet, and improved his hydration. He bought a device that tracked his heart rate variability each morning, and he began structuring his training around those numbers with the same discipline he had brought to everything. The HRV numbers were telling him to rest. He was resting. The resting was not producing the recovery the numbers suggested it should.

The feedback loop between effort and outcome had changed. He was beginning to recognize it, though not without considerable resistance. He used to be able to read his body during a session. A hard run felt hard, a recovery run felt easy, and he could trust those signals to mean something about what the next day would require. That reliable translation between effort and consequence had become unreliable.

He could finish a run that felt strong and still spend the following two days managing the consequences. He could no longer trust his own sense of how much was too much.

The sense and the consequence had come apart.

"I've always known how to push and how to back off," he said. "That's been automatic for twenty years. Now I genuinely don't know. I finish a session, and I have no idea what it's going to cost me."

He was not looking for permission to stop running. He was looking for an explanation of why running had stopped working. The question he had been asking for eighteen months, in the careful, disciplined way he approached every problem, was this: why is what I have always done no longer working?

The answer required understanding not what was wrong with his runs, but what was wrong with his recovery from them. And that required understanding something about the body's energy system that most fitness culture gets exactly backward.

Not Failure. Caution.

What was happening to David was not what most people assume is happening when recovery begins to fail. He was not running out of energy. He was running into a system that had become increasingly cautious about spending it. The body was not behaving as though the run itself was the problem. It was behaving as though recovery from the run could no longer be assumed.

The story most people were taught about mitochondria is incomplete. Energy production is one of their jobs. Adjusting that production to the conditions around them is another. They are not passive energy factories. They are responsive regulators within a much larger decision-making system.

Mitochondria continually respond to their cellular environment. They integrate molecular signals shaped by the nervous, immune, and hormonal systems, along with local conditions such as oxygen, nutrient availability, and the demands created by activity and recovery.

Those signals alter mitochondrial behavior in ways that are both logical and adaptive to the conditions within the cell. Together, they influence how energy is produced and used, how much reserve remains available, and how cellular resources are divided between immediate demand and subsequent repair.

David was not failing to produce energy during the run. He was failing to recover from the total physiologic demand the run created. The output was still available. The recovery required to make that output repeatable was not.

A system can have a long training history and adequate fuel available and still shift toward conservation if the surrounding conditions repeatedly interfere with complete recovery. This is the key distinction. The body is not failing to produce energy. It is becoming increasingly cautious about spending it because recovery has not yet proven itself reliable.

What conditions? The sustained threat response of an autonomic system that has remained in protective mode for months—the body still bracing for danger that has long since passed. The inflammatory activity of an immune system that has not fully resolved—symptoms that improve, then return, never quite disappearing completely. The degraded overnight repair that follows when circadian organization and restorative sleep have lost strength—nights that no longer deliver the patient back to themselves.

These lived patterns reflect the neuroendocrine, inflammatory, metabolic, and circadian signals to which cells and mitochondria are responding. Taken together, they create conditions in which complete recovery cannot yet be assumed. As the layers below begin to stabilize, those conditions change. The system gradually receives evidence that recovery can be trusted again.

This helps explain why interventions aimed primarily at increasing energy availability may produce incomplete or short-lived improvement when the conditions interfering with recovery remain unchanged. They may increase substrate availability or support parts of energy metabolism, but the system still encounters the same unresolved conditions: a nervous system preparing for danger, an immune system carrying unfinished work, and a recovery process that has not yet become reliable. The message remains the same. Conserve.

Not every person who struggles to recover after physical activity is struggling for the reasons described in this chapter. Some people struggle because their heart or lungs cannot adequately support the demands of physical activity. Others struggle because illness, anemia, medication effects, or other medical disorders have reduced their physical capacity in ways that require a different investigation. The pattern described here is different: a person who can still perform the activity but cannot reliably recover from it. The framework presented in this book is designed to help distinguish this pattern from others that require a different explanation. It does not replace appropriate medical evaluation when a different pattern is present.

Completing the Session Is Not the Same as Absorbing It

Many patients in Phase 4 describe the same set of observations. The battery never fully recharges. Good days arrive and then disappear without warning. Energy seems to be available—and yet does not seem to be usable, not in the way it once was.

The usual assumption is that the body has simply grown weaker, or that age has arrived. But weakness alone does not fully explain the pattern.

Think of cellular energy production as a freight train. The engine may have plenty of power. But if the maintenance crew has fallen behind on repairs, every trip leaves a little more wear than can be repaired before the next one begins. The train still runs. It still arrives. And the speed it holds today tells you nothing about how far behind the crew has fallen—though the crew is what determines whether the same trip can be made next week.

At the cellular level, these are genuinely different jobs. Producing energy is one. Repairing what the effort consumed is another. Keeping the system in condition to do both again is a third. These functions depend on overlapping systems but unfold through different processes and timelines, and a body can be performing the first well while falling steadily behind on the others.

Output and adaptation are not the same thing. A body can produce effort without adapting to it. It can complete a session, hit the targets, finish the distance, and simultaneously be accumulating a recovery debt it cannot pay. The session happened. The adaptation did not. And from the outside—even from the inside, during the session itself—there is no way to tell the difference.

This is the experience David was describing. The runs felt normal. He was finishing them. But finishing is not adapting. The adaptation—the physiologic response to the stimulus that makes the body stronger, more efficient, more resilient—requires a recovery phase that matches the demand. If recovery is able to complete the work the session created, the body adapts. If recovery is unable to complete that work, the body pays the cost of the session without receiving the full benefit. The next session begins from a system that has not finished recovering from the previous one. The debt accumulates.

Patients often describe this as never quite getting back to baseline. The day is decent. The night's sleep is decent. But the body never reaches the level of restoration it used to deliver routinely. Yesterday's effort is still being paid for tomorrow.

A body that can perform once but cannot recover to perform again is not adapting.

It is borrowing.

Completing the session is not the same as absorbing it. What the body can do once is not the same as what it can recover from repeatedly. That distinction is the entire content of Phase 4.

Why More Is Not the Answer

There is an intuition about fatigue and exercise that is so deeply embedded in fitness culture that it functions almost as a moral principle: if you are tired, push through. If your body is not responding, work harder. If the results are not coming, increase the load.

In a healthy system with adequate recovery capacity, this intuition is sometimes correct. Progressive overload—the systematic increase of demand over time—is a real mechanism for improvement. The body adapts to increasing demand. That is not wrong.

In a system where the recovery capacity is insufficient, this intuition is not just unhelpful. It is actively counterproductive. And the damage is not always visible immediately.

The pattern goes like this. The person increases the load because the previous load seemed manageable. The session completes. The session felt fine, or even good—adrenaline and accumulated training base can support output that exceeds what the recovery system can actually process. Two days later, the fatigue is significantly worse than expected. The person concludes they pushed too hard. They reduce the load, take a recovery week, and return to training feeling somewhat better. They push again. The pattern repeats. Each cycle extracts a slightly larger recovery cost. The good periods get shorter. The crash periods get longer.

This is not deconditioning. It is not weakness. It is not aging. It is a system whose recovery capacity cannot keep pace with the demand being placed on it. And because the signals of recovery failure are delayed, the system is often pushed harder rather than protected.

In Phase 4, the most important consequence often arrives forty-eight hours after the effort that caused it. This is the interpretive trap that makes the pattern so difficult to recognize and so easy to worsen. The session ends feeling successful. Because nothing goes wrong immediately, the session gets classified internally as managed. The person goes to bed that night without a clear signal that something was miscalculated. The following morning feels acceptable. And then Tuesday arrives, or Wednesday, with a fatigue that seems disproportionate to anything that happened—and gets attributed to poor sleep, or a stressful day, or something in the diet, or simple bad luck. The original effort and its consequence never get connected, because the timing between them is too long for ordinary cause-and-effect thinking to bridge.

Consider a patient who has rested for two weeks, feels genuinely better, and returns to training—cautiously, they think. The sessions feel manageable. Energy is higher than it has been in months. They increase the load slightly. Five days later, the fatigue is worse than before the rest period began. The sleep has deteriorated. The morning heart rate is elevated. They cannot identify a single session that caused it because none of the individual sessions felt excessive. The cause was the pattern—the cumulative demand that never felt excessive session by session while quietly exceeding the recovery system's actual capacity.

This is why intelligent, disciplined people so often get worse by doing exactly what used to work. Not through laziness or denial or lack of effort. But because the feedback timing itself is distorted. They push harder in response to a delayed signal they have misread. They interpret the delayed fatigue as evidence that they are deconditioned and need more training, not less. They increase the load precisely when the system is already in recovery debt. And the debt grows.

The answer is not to stop exercising. Exercise is not the problem. Demand without sufficient recovery is the problem. The distinction is everything. A system that cannot currently recover from five sessions per week can recover from three. A system that cannot recover from sixty-minute sessions can recover from thirty-minute ones. The goal is not less activity. The goal is finding the level at which recovery actually completes—and starting there.

The Repeatability Principle

Of all the clinical concepts that change how patients understand their own recovery, the one that produces the most consistent and dramatic shift is what I call the repeatability principle. It is simple to state. It is genuinely difficult to accept. And it is the most important single measure of progress available in Phase 4.

The principle is this.

A single good session means almost nothing. What matters is whether you can do it again.

In conventional fitness thinking, a good workout is evidence of sustainable capacity. Completing a demanding session can tell you something meaningful about current performance. That logic holds true in a regulated system with adequate recovery infrastructure—the ability to recover from one session before the next.

In a body that does not yet recover reliably between sessions, a good session is not evidence of sustainable capacity. It is evidence of what the body can do today. The relevant question is not whether you completed the session. It is whether you can complete the same session in two or three days, and again two or three days after that, and whether the quality of your recovery across those repeated exposures stays consistent or degrades.

If recovery degrades—if the second session leaves you more fatigued than the first, if the third session produces a crash, if a week of consistent activity is followed by a week of setback—then the demand exceeded the recovery capacity. Not dramatically, perhaps. But the compounding is real, and its consequences are the pattern many people in Phase 4 recognize: good weeks followed by crashes, progress followed by regression, effort that costs more than it builds.

This can eventually become visible in performance as well. The weightlifter lifts less. The pitcher throws slower. The runner finds that the same pace costs more than it used to.

One good session is data. Consistent good recovery across repeated sessions is progress. The distinction between these two things is everything in Phase 4, and confusing them is the most common and most costly mistake in energy recovery.

The practical implication is demanding in its simplicity: reduce the load until you find the level at which recovery is functionally complete before the next session. Not mostly complete. Not good enough to continue. Functionally complete means that the second session produces the same quality of recovery as the first, and the third the same as the second, across a sustained period.

This instruction meets significant resistance in almost every patient who hears it. The disciplined person—the runner, the athlete, the high-performer who has always believed that consistency and effort produce results—experiences a reduction in training load as a form of failure. It feels like regression. It feels like giving in. It activates something that is not just physical but identity-level: the belief that doing less means becoming less. That belief is understandable. It is also, in Phase 4, precisely the belief that is preventing improvement.

That level is the adaptive window. It is the level from which genuine, sustainable improvement becomes possible. Most people in Phase 4 are operating significantly above it, which is why their effort produces so little lasting adaptation.

The adaptive window is not failure. It is the starting point.

How do you know when recovery is functionally complete? The markers are specific and observable. Morning heart rate at or below your personal resting baseline. Energy on the day after a session that is not meaningfully worse than the day before. Sleep quality that does not degrade in the days following activity. The ability to repeat the effort without increasing symptoms. These are not elaborate metrics. They are the body's own report on whether the last demand was absorbed.

The Recovery Protocol

Reducing the load is one half of meeting the body where it is. The other half is what happens in the thirty minutes after the session ends. Most people treat the end of the workout as the end of the work. In Phase 4, the consequences of this mistake are often delayed enough that patients never recognize it as a mistake at all.

The thirty minutes after the session are, at this layer of the sequence, as important as the session itself. More precisely, they determine whether the session is completed. The recovery protocol is the second half of the therapeutic intervention—the operational version of what the chapter has been teaching all along: completing the session is not the same as absorbing it.

Exercise activates the sympathetic nervous system—the body's accelerator—which is appropriate and necessary during the session. Mobilization is not the problem. It is what the effort requires. In a well-regulated system, the shift back from accelerator to brake happens on its own once the effort ends. In Phase 4, that shift often does not happen as quickly or as completely as it should. The accelerator stays partly engaged longer than intended. The patient usually notices this without recognizing what it is: the wired feeling that does not fade, the heart rate that stays elevated for an hour after the run, the appetite that does not arrive, the sense of carrying the workout into the rest of the day. The problem is not activation itself. It is that the activation does not end when the demand does.

Immediately after the session—before eating, before showering, before anything else—lie on your back with your legs elevated. Against a wall, couch, or whatever is available. Five to ten minutes. Elevating the legs reduces the immediate circulatory demand on the heart and gives the body a low-demand position from which to begin leaving the exercise state. The patient who has been doing this for a few weeks often notices the wired feeling that used to last for hours starting to fade within minutes.

While in that position, begin the breathing practice from Chapter 3. Four to six seconds in, four to six seconds out, nasal breathing, nothing forced. Slow, unforced breathing gives the body another cue that the period of demand has ended—one of the few levers a person can reach directly, without having to decide their way into calm.

After the breathing—not before, not during—eat twenty-five to thirty grams of protein, keeping the entire recovery sequence within the first thirty minutes after the session. The sequencing matters. First help the body end the demand. Then provide the materials recovery requires. Beginning the shift out of exertion before eating allows the body to begin leaving the exercise state before asking it to begin digesting a meal.

Add electrolytes alongside the protein. Recovery depends not only on calories and amino acids but also on fluid and mineral balance. Exercise can increase those needs through sweating and fluid shifts, particularly during longer, harder, or hotter sessions. In Phase 4, thoughtful electrolyte replacement should be treated as part of the recovery sequence rather than an optional extra.

Legs up, breathing, then protein and electrolytes, in that sequence. Thirty minutes. Every session. The body receives the stimulus of exercise. The recovery sequence supplies the lower-demand conditions in which that stimulus can be processed. And the next session has a better chance of beginning from a body that has recovered rather than one still paying for the last demand.

The Body Learns the Way Back

There is a deeper reason the recovery protocol matters, beyond its effect on heart rate, breathing, circulation, and nourishment. Every session contains two kinds of training. The first is the physical demand itself—the run, the lift, the effort. The second is quieter, and most people never notice it: the pattern the body experiences in the minutes after the demand ends.

A regulated nervous system is not one that stays calm. It is one that can mobilize when demand requires it and return when the demand is over. The accelerator is supposed to engage. The question is whether the body can find its way back afterward—and in Phase 4, the way back is often what has been lost.

We usually think of safety as a fact about the world: nothing dangerous is happening. The body treats safety differently. It treats it as a physiologic condition—something read from the state of the body itself, not concluded from the situation. And the two do not always agree. A person can know, with complete intellectual certainty, that the workout is over, while the body goes on behaving as though effort is still required. The mind knows the session has ended before the body does.

Polyvagal Theory offers one framework for understanding this. Within that framework, the felt sense of safety reflects autonomic states that quiet defensive reactions and make restoration, digestion, growth, and connection more available—a shift that happens beneath conscious awareness, which is why it cannot simply be decided. When defensive mobilization persists, resources remain organized around meeting demand. When that state resolves, the body can begin returning toward biological equilibrium.

Healing depends not only on what the body experiences. It also depends on what the body comes to expect.

This is the same principle Chapter 5 named from a different direction: a nervous system that cannot trust the environment cannot invest in repair. There, the environment was the whole life—safety, rhythm, relationship. Here it is something much smaller and more immediate. Each time a session of demand ends in a calm, nourished, unhurried recovery, the body is given another experience of what tends to follow effort.

For the autonomic nervous system, consistency creates predictability. Predictability does not guarantee safety—a harmful pattern can be perfectly predictable—but a demand that reliably ends in restoration creates a repeated pattern in which effort has an ending, and the ending is not another emergency. Over many repetitions the sequence becomes familiar: demand, completion, downshift, nourishment, restoration. The body becomes less likely to carry the effort forward as though it has not ended.

This is one of the ways the adaptive window begins to expand. Not force. The adaptive window does not widen because the body is forced to tolerate more. It widens because the body repeatedly completes what it is already being asked to tolerate. Repeated overshoot teaches the opposite lesson. Repeated successful recovery teaches the body that demand does not have to end in recovery debt.

The same logic runs underneath much of what this book has recommended. A consistent wake time. Meals at predictable hours. Morning light. Recovery days that are genuinely restorative rather than merely less demanding. None of these are only about their immediate mechanical effect. Each is a repeated experience in which the body is given a reliable pattern to organize around—which is why small, unglamorous, repeated interventions often produce more stable change than dramatic ones.

This is why the recovery protocol is more than a set of post-workout techniques. Legs elevated, slow breathing, protein, electrolytes—across sessions, these create a repeated transition from effort into restoration. Any single session matters little. The pattern across sessions is the point.

The body does not need a life without demand. It needs repeated evidence that demand will be followed by recovery.

Foundation Work You Can Do Now

David was not someone who needed to stop running. His system was not fully depleted. It was operating with insufficient recovery permission—capable of activity but not recovering from it efficiently enough for that activity to remain adaptive.

The change he needed was not to stop. It was to change what he was measuring. He had been measuring performance—pace, distance, effort level, the feeling during the session. None of those measures captured what actually determined whether his running was helping or harming him. The correct measure was recovery quality: what happened in the twenty-four to forty-eight hours after the session.

Begin measuring recovery, not performance.

After any physical activity, observe what happens over the next forty-eight hours. How does your sleep compare with baseline? Is your energy the following day better, equivalent, or worse than it was before the activity? Are symptoms such as fatigue, brain fog, digestive reactivity, or joint sensitivity elevated above their usual baseline? These observations, accumulated across sessions, will tell you more about where you currently are in the adaptive sequence than any performance metric.

If the recovery observations are consistently negative—if activity is followed by worse sleep, lower energy, or elevated symptoms—reduce the load. Not permanently. To the level at which recovery normalizes.

That level is your current adaptive window, and it is the level from which genuine, repeatable progress becomes possible.

Apply the recovery protocol after every session, regardless of how brief or easy the session felt. The protocol is not a reward for difficult workouts. It is how the body learns that demand will be followed by recovery.

The most important shift in Phase 4 is learning to read a different signal as progress. For most disciplined people, progress has always felt like more—more distance, more weight, more sessions, more output. Phase 4 asks for something that feels like its opposite: less load, more observation, and a willingness to recognize improved recovery as progress even when performance has not yet improved.

Scaling down is not regression. Finding your adaptive window is not giving up. For many people, it is the first genuinely honest conversation they have had with their body in months or years—one in which they are finally asking what it can recover from rather than what it can perform once. That reframe is not a concession. It is a correction. And it is the correction that makes everything above it possible.

The adaptive window is not a permanent ceiling. As upstream conditions improve—the nervous system stabilizes, immune activation resolves, and circadian amplitude is restored—the capacity for recovery expands. Sessions that are currently beyond the window will eventually be within it. The body will demonstrate this not through a feeling but through a pattern: the recovery holds, the morning heart rate stays at baseline, the following day is not worse than the day before. Progress in Phase 4 looks like that. Not like the feeling during the session. Like the consistency of what happens after it.

David implemented both changes. He reduced his running to three sessions per week, each slightly shorter than his previous standard. He added the recovery protocol. And he changed, fundamentally, what he tracked. He stopped treating pace and mileage as the measures that mattered. He started tracking morning heart rate, sleep quality, and next-day energy. Within six weeks, for the first time in eighteen months, the pattern was consistent. The sessions were producing recovery that held. The following days were not worse than the days before.

He told me the moment he noticed it was not a good run. It was a Tuesday morning, the day after a Monday session, when he looked at his HRV, and the number matched how he actually felt. Not elevated. Not crashing. Just baseline—exactly where it should be. He had not been waiting for that number to tell him he had overdone it. For eighteen months that had been the shape of his mornings: check the data, calculate the cost, adjust the day accordingly. That Tuesday he had checked the data and there was nothing to adjust. The session had simply been absorbed. He stood in the kitchen for a moment, not quite sure what to do with the absence of the calculation.

"I thought I was just getting old," he told me. "Like the body just stops responding the way it used to. I thought I had to accept that."

He paused.

"But it wasn't aging. The sequence was wrong. The body was right."

The next layer is the one most patients think of first because the loss of strength, resilience, and structural capacity is the most visible. But before the body can become stronger, it must demonstrate something more important: that recovery can remain stable as demand increases. We will look at why so many attempts to rebuild fail, why progress often disappears as quickly as it arrives, and why strength returns most reliably when recovery remains in control of the process.

CHAPTER NINE

Rebuilding

"The body is never resisting greater physical capacity. It is waiting until it has the biology to support it."
—Marcus Ettinger, DC

Nadia

Her name is Nadia. She was forty-seven years old, a physical therapist—a detail that mattered in a specific and painful way. She had spent her career helping other people rebuild strength and function after injury and illness. She understood progressive loading, tissue adaptation, recovery windows, and the physiology of exercise response better than most of my patients. She understood, intellectually, exactly how rebuilding was supposed to work. What she could not understand was why her own body was not responding.

She had been ill for four years with a condition that combined significant fatigue, immune dysregulation, and what she described as a "catastrophic loss of physical strength and endurance." She had gone from someone who routinely lifted and transferred patients, who exercised regularly and without consequence, who thought of physical capability as a stable and fundamental part of who she was—to someone who had begun calculating the recovery cost of activities she once performed without a second thought.

She described this loss with a precision few people outside the clinical world could have. She knew exactly which muscles had weakened. She knew the functional benchmarks she could no longer meet. She could describe, in clinical language, exactly what the deconditioning looked like and what rehabilitation should theoretically produce. And that clinical literacy made her situation harder to bear—because she understood, better than most, how far she had fallen and how large the gap was between where she was and where she needed to be.

What she had lost was not only strength. What she had lost was the ability to trust her body's response to effort.

Before the illness, exertion had been reliable. She pushed; the body responded. She loaded; the tissue adapted. She rested; she recovered. The feedback loop between effort and outcome was something she had counted on so consistently that she had stopped noticing—the way you stop noticing a floor that has always held you.

The illness had removed that floor. And even after the worst of the acute phase had passed, the floor had not returned in the way she expected.

She had begun to hesitate before physical tasks she would previously have performed without thought. Not because she was uncertain of the technique—she knew the technique. She could no longer predict what the task would cost. Would a session of moderate exercise produce normal fatigue, or would it produce extended depletion that had once turned a single workout into a week-long setback? Would she recover overnight, or would the next two days be consumed by managing a crash? She had begun doing mental calculations before movement—assessing risk, estimating cost, deciding whether the activity was worth the uncertain consequence. Exercise, which had always been a source of capability and control, had become something she approached carefully, the way you approach a surface that might or might not hold your weight.

There was a specific professional humiliation in this. She worked with patients in the early stages of their own rebuilding—patients who were scared, uncertain, and needed someone to demonstrate that recovery was possible. She gave them that. She talked them through their fear of pushing harder. She showed them how the body adapts to progressive demand, how soreness resolves, how strength returns. And she did it while privately managing her own recovery, which was not going the way she was telling her patients theirs would go. She had watched patients she was treating rebuild faster than she was. She had wondered, more than once, whether she was overlooking something obvious.

"I understand the physiology," she told me. "I can explain exactly why adaptation should be happening. And it isn't. And I don't know what to do with the gap between what I know and what is actually happening."

By the time she came to see me, the worst of the acute illness had passed. She had stabilized. Her energy, while not what it had been, was more reliable. Her sleep had improved. Her immune reactivity had reduced significantly. She had earned her way, carefully and methodically, to the point where rebuilding felt both possible and urgent. She had begun a resistance training program six months before our first appointment. She started conservatively, progressed slowly, and monitored her response. Yet she had hit a wall she could not explain.

Her strength was improving, but slowly. Painfully slowly. Her recovery from training sessions was longer than it should have been given the modest loads she was using. And she had a persistent sense of uncertainty—a clinical intuition that years of practice develops—that something was still not quite right at a level the training itself could not address.

"I feel like I'm building on sand," she told me. "Like the work is going in, but it's not sticking the way it should."

That is the most precise description of what happens when rebuilding is initiated before all the sub-processes of the structural layer are in place.

Building on Sand

A pattern of failed rebuilding can appear in patients who begin structural work before the lower layers are fully stable. The pattern has nothing to do with effort.

Strength gains arrive and then plateau earlier than expected. Progress that felt real in the first few weeks stalls before it consolidates. Soreness from modest sessions lasts two or three days rather than one. Training tolerance fluctuates in ways that are genuinely confusing—a session that felt manageable this week produces significant depletion next week at the same load. Good weeks do not become stable weeks. They become the peaks of a cycle in which effort extracts more than it returns, and the gap between what was spent and what was recovered accumulates until a crash resets the progress.

In this pattern, the body can produce effort before it can sustain adaptation.

Completing a session is not the same as adapting to it. A workout can be finished successfully while the rebuilding it was meant to stimulate never fully takes hold.

Not all rebuilding difficulty or failed physical adaptation reflects Phase 5 instability, and some patterns—including primary musculoskeletal pathology, neuromuscular conditions, structural injury, and other medical issues—require their own assessment. The framework here interprets a specific and recognizable physiologic rebuilding pattern within the EFP sequence. It does not replace clinical evaluation.

The work goes in. The results do not stick.

The reason is not in the session itself.

Recovery Is Not Rebuilding

Many patients reach a point in their recovery where something genuinely changes. Sleep deepens. Energy stabilizes. Symptoms that defined their days for years begin to recede. They tolerate activity more reliably. The decline has stopped. By any reasonable measure, recovery is working. Yet they describe themselves with a precision that contains both progress and limitation. They feel better. They are not yet restored. They have stopped getting worse. They have not yet returned. Recovery is happening. Something else is not.

Recovery and rebuilding are not the same thing, but they are stages of the same process: healing. Each has a distinct biologic job, and those jobs happen in sequence—the body cannot do the second until it has finished the first. Recovery restores function—the ability to do what an ordinary day requires without depletion. A person who has recovered can do what an ordinary day asks of them—they can work, sleep, eat, move, and tolerate the demands their life routinely produces. That is what recovery delivers, and after years of being unable to count on it, the reliability itself is a profound restoration.

Rebuilding restores reserve—the underlying capacity the body draws on when ordinary demands change, when illness returns, and when the day asks for more. Rebuilding restores the margin—the buffer between what the day requires and what the body has available to give. A rebuilt body has reserve left over after meeting the day's needs. The difference shows up when life stops cooperating. A difficult week no longer creates a month-long setback. An illness no longer wipes out months of progress. The unexpected costs what it should cost—no more.

This is why so many patients in Phase 5 describe themselves with a kind of double awareness. They know they have improved. They know it in their sleep, in their energy, and in their tolerance for the demands of an ordinary day. And they also know that they are not yet fully restored. The body has stopped declining. The body has not yet rebuilt. These are different milestones, and the patient who has crossed the first one is right to notice that they have not yet crossed the second.

The body itself shifts its question at this point. For years, the body has been asking whether recovery can be trusted. Whether demand can be safely produced. Whether the system can return to a state in which effort and outcome reliably connect. That question has now been answered. The body knows recovery is possible. It is asking a different question now, one that the chapters before this could not yet pose. Not "Can recovery happen?" but "Is there enough capacity available to rebuild?" The rest of this chapter explores what the body needs before it can answer that question with yes.

Recovery allows participation in life. Rebuilding allows the body to expand back into it.

The Fear That Develops

In the previous chapter, we saw how repeated successful recovery teaches the body that demand can once again be trusted. The same learning process also works in the opposite direction. Repeated failed rebuilding teaches the body that exertion itself carries risk.

When the body has repeatedly responded to exercise with unexpected and disproportionate consequences—a session that seemed reasonable produces a crash that lasts days, an increase in load is followed by a week of regression, and effort and outcome no longer connect reliably—the body learns something. Not consciously. Physiologically. It learns that exertion is a source of risk rather than a pathway toward greater improvement.

This is a recalibration of the nervous system's assessment of what exertion means. The nervous system has received repeated evidence that physical demand produces unpredictable consequences. It responds to that evidence by lowering the threshold at which exertion is flagged as a potential threat. Movement that was previously unremarkable begins to generate an anticipatory stress response. The body starts preparing for a cost before the work has even begun. The approach to exercise becomes tentative, calculating, and hypervigilant in a way that was never there before.

The person who has been through multiple rebuilding failures begins doing the same calculations Nadia described—assessing the risk of each physical task, estimating how long recovery might take, and deciding whether the effort is worth what may follow. They may begin avoiding activities they once associated with capability and freedom. Not because they have consciously decided to avoid them. Because the body has learned that those activities carry uncertain costs. The nervous system naturally favors actions whose consequences are predictable. When exertion no longer produces predictable outcomes, the nervous system becomes more cautious.

Understanding this matters because it changes how rebuilding must be approached. A nervous system that has learned to treat exertion as risk cannot be successfully retrained through more exertion. It needs to accumulate evidence, through repeated successful recovery, that demand can be followed by completion. That the cost can be predicted. That the floor will hold.

Capacity expands only after recovery becomes reliable. Until the nervous system has reliable evidence that recovery can be counted on, it will resist greater demand by making activity feel more costly and exertion something to protect against rather than adapt to.

The Three Jobs of Rebuilding

The structural repair layer of the hierarchy—Phase 5, the rebuilding of strength, resilience, and physical capacity—is not a single process. It is a sequence of three processes that must occur in order, the same way the layers of the hierarchy must occur in order.

The first process is the stabilization of energy production. The mitochondria must consistently generate enough energy to support daily function without depleting the system. Not peak performance—consistent, reliable function that does not degrade under ordinary daily demands.

The second process is the recovery of resilience. Resilience is the ability to be stressed—by activity, by demand, and by the ordinary challenges of a full life—and to recover from that stress within a reasonable and consistent timeframe. Not the total absence of fatigue after exertion. The reliable return to baseline within forty-eight hours of resuming normal activity.

The third process is structural rebuilding. The progressive loading of muscle, connective tissue, and bone that stimulates the specific repair and growth signals required to restore, maintain, and expand physical capacity.

Patients most often attempt the third process first because it is the most visible part of recovery—the part that feels like you're doing something. It is the part you can see in the mirror, measure in the gym, and feel progressing from week to week. But without the two layers beneath it, the rebuilding rarely stabilizes for long. That is the pattern Nadia had lived through before we changed the sequence.

Each of these three processes depends on the one before it. Structural rebuilding requires resilience, because rebuilding generates tissue breakdown that the recovery system must repair. Resilience requires stable energy production, because the recovery process is itself energetically expensive. Stable energy production requires everything below it in the hierarchy—the nervous system foundation, the immune regulation, the circadian repair—that the preceding chapters have addressed.

The reason premature rebuilding produces regression is not that the body is incapable of rebuilding. It is that the body is protecting itself. Rebuilding generates a repair demand that the system cannot meet when the energy and recovery infrastructure beneath it is not yet sufficient. The body is asked to repair more than it can process, and the deficit accumulates until the system reduces demand to restore stability.

The body is never resisting greater physical capacity. It is waiting until it has the biology to support it.

Permission vs Capacity

Patients who reach this phase of recovery often arrive at the same question: if recovery is finally working, why isn't rebuilding? They have done the work of stabilizing energy, restoring sleep, reducing immune reactivity, and rebuilding the conditions that allow ordinary life to be lived again. Recovery is no longer the question. And yet, when they begin to expand their lives—to take on more activity, to ask the body for more than the day routinely requires—something does not respond the way it should. There is a reason. And it has nothing to do with effort.

Rebuilding requires more than the right signal. It requires capacity—the body's ability to support the work of rebuilding once it has been initiated. The signal can be present, the protocol can be correct, the effort can be appropriate—and the rebuilding will still proceed only as fast as the body can support it. When that capacity is sufficient, rebuilding proceeds at the rate the signal asks for. When any part of it is incomplete, rebuilding stalls—regardless of the signal.

This distinction is the architectural pivot point of the recovery sequence. Chapter 8 was largely about permission—the body's willingness to produce energy, to allow demand to be generated, to lift the protective restrictions that had been holding the system at a reduced level of function. Chapter 9 is largely about capacity—the body's ability to support the work of rebuilding once permission has been granted. Permission allows the work to begin. Capacity determines how much work can be done. These are different mechanisms operating in sequence, and they require different conditions to be addressed.

A body that has restored permission but not capacity behaves in a recognizable way. It can begin the work of rebuilding. It cannot complete it at the rate the rebuilding would otherwise proceed.

Effort produces the signal. Capacity shapes the response. The signal may arrive at a body that cannot yet support all of what it is asking for.

Rebuilding proceeds at the rate of whichever part of the system is most depleted. This is the principle of the limiting factor. Anyone who has slept ten hours and still woken exhausted knows the feeling—the missing ingredient was never sleep.

A body with enough signal but too few materials rebuilds at the rate of the materials. A body with enough signal and materials but unable to recover between sessions rebuilds at the rate of the recovery. Adding more of what is not limiting produces no acceleration. The work proceeds at the speed of the slowest part of the process.

The signal tells the body where to build. Capacity determines how much building can occur. Permission allows the work to begin. Capacity determines how far it can proceed.

The Construction Problem

The nervous system opens the construction site. The body still needs bricks. This is the part of rebuilding that signal alone cannot solve, and the part that catches most patients by surprise.

Permission grants access to the work. Capacity makes the work possible. But the work itself is physical—the construction of new tissue, the laying down of new fiber, the repair of structures that have been depleted over the years of illness. Construction requires materials. The most precisely timed mechanical signal, arriving in a perfectly regulated body, can only direct what is already there. It cannot create from nothing. Where there are no materials, there is no construction—regardless of how clearly the body has been told where to build.

Nadia had spent years trying to get her body to allow rebuilding. She had done the work of restoring permission—the sleep, the regulation, the long arc of stabilizing the systems that had been holding her body in protection. She had assumed that once permission was granted, rebuilding would naturally follow. What she had not realized was that allowing rebuilding and supplying rebuilding were different problems. The body she had worked so carefully to free had been waiting for materials that were simply not there in sufficient quantity.

The materials are not exotic. They are the raw materials the body uses to construct biological tissue—protein, minerals, water, and the cellular building blocks that every repair process requires. The body is asking for enough of them to complete the work the signal is initiating. When those raw materials are present in sufficient quantity, rebuilding proceeds. When they are not, the signal arrives at a body that cannot fulfill what it is being asked to do.

The body can build with ordinary materials. It cannot build without them.

There is an assumption worth bringing to light. Most people who eat what they consider a healthy diet assume the materials are present. Often they are. But sometimes they are not, and the gap is rarely obvious from the inside—a diet that feels adequate can still fall short of what active rebuilding demands, and the shortfall shows up not as hunger but as rebuilding that stalls for no visible reason. The materials are worth verifying rather than assuming. That can begin with an honest look at what the body is actually being given each day and, when the picture remains unclear, with objective evaluation rather than continued assumption. The body builds from what is available, not from what we believe is available.

What the Body Is Actually Trying to Do

Structural rebuilding is not simply about getting stronger. It is the body's final act of returning to full physiologic self-sufficiency—the restoration of the physical reserves that allow a person to live an ordinary life without constantly managing their energy budget.

Healthy skeletal muscle is far more than tissue that produces movement. It is one of the body's largest metabolic organs, helping regulate blood glucose, store energy, and produce signaling proteins that communicate with the brain, immune system, liver, and cardiovascular system. Just as importantly, it serves as one of the body's greatest physiologic reserves during illness, stress, and recovery. When muscle mass is lost—as it is, consistently, in the context of chronic illness—the loss is not just physical. It is a reduction in the body's overall metabolic and immunologic reserve.

This is why patients often continue feeling physically fragile long after the acute illness itself has stabilized—the structural reserve that allows ordinary life to feel ordinary has not yet been rebuilt.

Rebuilding that reserve is the final act of the hierarchy for a reason. It is the most energetically and hormonally expensive process in the recovery sequence. It requires abundant protein, sufficient anabolic signaling, consistent mechanical stimulus, and a recovery infrastructure capable of handling the repair load generated by progressive resistance training. None of those requirements can be met while the layers below are still unstable.

But when the layers below are stable—when the nervous system has restored its regulatory flexibility, the immune system has reduced its inflammatory burden, the circadian clock is generating the growth hormone pulse that helps drive tissue repair during slow-wave sleep, and the mitochondria are producing energy reliably enough to support both daily function and recovery—the body rebuilds with a speed and consistency that surprises patients who have been stuck for years.

The body knows how to rebuild. It has always known. What it needed was the conditions under which rebuilding is safe. Those conditions are what the body has been waiting for all along.

The Mechanical Signal and What It Requires

Before we discuss what Nadia needed, I want to explain something about mechanical loading that is not widely understood outside of sports science and physical medicine—something that will change how you think about resistance training.

When muscle tissue is subjected to mechanical load—as it is during resistance training—a cascade of cellular events occurs that extends far beyond simple muscle fatigue and repair. The body translates that mechanical stimulus into intracellular signaling pathways. When combined with adequate amino acid availability, these pathways stimulate protein synthesis—the process of building new proteins that repair and strengthen muscle tissue over time.

This is the adaptive process of resistance training. The restoration of functional tissue, the recovery of metabolic reserve, and the rebuilding of the physiologic capacity that chronic illness has eroded.

But this process requires specific conditions. It requires adequate protein—particularly the amino acid leucine, which is especially abundant in animal protein and serves as one of the primary nutritional triggers for protein synthesis. It requires a hormonal environment that supports anabolism—particularly growth hormone, released in a circadian-timed pulse during slow-wave sleep, and its downstream mediator, IGF-1.

And it requires something that is easy to overlook and difficult to shortcut.

It requires inflammation to be low enough for rebuilding to proceed. When inflammation is high, acutely or chronically, the body activates competing pathways that work against muscle growth—pathways that not only block rebuilding but also accelerate the breakdown of the muscle that is already there.

This last condition is the critical one. The background immune activation that earlier chapters have been addressing is one of the primary drivers of muscle loss in chronic illness. The body is receiving two competing instructions at the same time: one directs resources toward rebuilding, the other toward defense. When the defensive signal is stronger—as it is when inflammation is high—the net result is the progressive loss of muscle that patients experience as physical diminishment.

Resistance training provides the mechanical signal that initiates rebuilding. Whether that rebuilding proceeds depends on the biologic conditions surrounding the signal.

This is why rebuilding must follow immune stabilization. Not as an arbitrary sequencing preference, but because the cellular machinery of rebuilding requires an inflammatory environment that has been sufficiently reduced to permit it to operate. Without that reduction, resistance training produces a stimulus that the body cannot fully respond to—and the result is exactly what Nadia described: work going in, results not sticking.

The Missing Third

When I examined Nadia's recovery protocol, I found what I see in a large proportion of patients who are doing the right things at this layer but not getting the results they should: she was missing the third condition.

Her protein intake was adequate. Her training program was well-designed. But one of the conditions required for rebuilding had not yet fully re-established itself. Her sleep was better than it had been, and recovery was clearly improving, but the circadian system that coordinates many of the body's overnight repair processes was still stabilizing.

She was asking the body to rebuild before the physiology that supports rebuilding had fully re-established itself.

She was training into a hormonal environment that was not yet fully supportive of the adaptation. The mechanical stimulus was appropriate. The protein was present. But as we saw in the previous section, much of the overnight rebuilding signal depends on a fully restored circadian rhythm. Hers was still consolidating. The conditions that allow effort to become lasting adaptation were not yet consistently present.

The solution was not to train harder or to change her program. It was to continue the circadian restoration work—the morning light, the consistent timing, the evening disengagement—with renewed attention to the specific goal of restoring slow-wave sleep depth. And to adjust her training schedule to align with the times of day when her hormonal environment was most favorable to adaptation: morning and early afternoon, when the body's natural rhythms support rebuilding, rather than late afternoon or evening when the clock is beginning its shift toward overnight repair.

Three months later, her strength gains had doubled their previous rate. Same program. Same protein. Same effort. Different hormonal environment. The work that had been going in and not sticking was now sticking—because the conditions that allowed it to take hold had finally been fully established.

She told me the first sign of it was not a training session. It was a Saturday morning when she carried the groceries in from the car without running the calculation first. Not the weight of the bags, not the number of trips, and not the cost against the afternoon. She had simply picked them up and carried them in. Only afterward did she notice this—standing in the kitchen, bags on the counter—when she realized the floor had been there the whole time and she had stopped testing it.

Rebuilding Is Not Linear

Structural rebuilding rarely progresses in a straight line. Strength improves, plateaus, and improves again. Recovery expands, contracts, and expands again. Without understanding this pattern, patients often abandon rebuilding efforts that are actually working.

Adaptation follows the same pattern. Some weeks will feel like genuine forward progress. Others will feel like regression—reduced tolerance, slower recovery, sessions that produce more fatigue than the previous week's equivalent. This is not a sign that something has gone wrong. It is a sign that the body is running its adaptation cycle, which naturally includes periods of consolidation—times when the body is catching up to the work that has already been done. From the inside, these periods often feel as though nothing is happening.

What matters is not the trajectory of individual sessions or individual weeks. It is the trend across months. A patient who is stronger at six months than at three months, and stronger at nine months than at six, is making genuine progress—even if there were weeks in each of those periods that felt like setbacks. The body's adaptation to progressive loading is measured in months, not weeks. And the fluctuations within that arc are not evidence of failure. They are what rebuilding looks like.

The practical implication is important: do not make decisions about your rebuilding program based on how this week compares to last week. Make them based on how this month compares to the month before. If the trend is upward over a longer arc, the program is working. If the trend is flat or declining over several months despite consistent effort and adequate recovery, that is the signal to reassess—not a bad week.

Foundation Work You Can Do Now

The practical guidance for this chapter is different from the guidance in the preceding chapters. The earlier practices—breathing, nature exposure, routine anchoring, light protocols, meal timing, and recovery protocol—are appropriate regardless of where you are in the recovery process. They address layers of the hierarchy that are relevant across the entire arc of chronic illness.

Resistance training for structural rebuilding is appropriate only when the lower layers are sufficiently stable to support it. And only you—in collaboration with the practitioners working with you—can make that assessment for your specific situation. What I can offer here are the principles that govern when rebuilding is likely to be productive and what it requires to be so.

The first principle: do not begin progressive resistance training while energy production is still unreliable and recovery from ordinary activity is still incomplete. The criterion from Chapter 8 applies here too: the system must be able to perform and recover from ordinary activity consistently before the additional repair demand of resistance training is introduced.

The second principle: when you begin, begin with less than feels necessary.

This instruction will feel wrong to almost everyone who follows it. The person who has spent months or years losing physical capacity does not experience restraint as wisdom. They experience it as more waiting. More time passing while the body they remember remains inaccessible. The impulse to increase the load—to do more, to prove that recovery is real, to accumulate visible evidence that the work is producing something. It is not impatience—it is the reasonable response of a person who has been ill for a long time and who needs to know that the direction has genuinely changed.

Understanding this does not make restraint easier. But it reframes what restraint is. The person who begins with less than feels necessary is not avoiding progress. They are protecting the conditions under which progress becomes durable. Every session completed within the adaptive window is a session that builds the evidence the nervous system needs: that demand can be followed by recovery, that the floor will hold, and that the body can be trusted again with increasing load. That evidence accumulates. Gradually, the adaptive window expands. Sessions that were previously beyond it are eventually within it. The restraint was not the obstacle. It was the mechanism.

Nadia described this, early in her rebuilding, as the hardest part of the entire recovery sequence. The waiting while doing less than she believed she could do. "I kept thinking I was wasting time," she said. "I wasn't. I was learning what my right amount was. And that was the part that had been missing."

The rebuilding signal requires only a fraction of the load that produces fatigue in a well-trained athlete. In a system recovering from chronic illness, even modest loads produce a meaningful mechanical stimulus. The question is not whether the stimulus is sufficient. The question is whether the system can recover from it completely before the next session.

The third principle: protein is not optional. Rebuilding requires raw materials, and protein is the primary raw material from which new tissue is constructed. As a general rule, aim for approximately 0.8 grams of protein per pound of body weight each day while rebuilding, distributed across multiple meals. That post-session protein intake is one of the easiest ways to meet this daily target, while supplying amino acids when the rebuilding signal has just been generated. Without adequate protein, the mechanical signal cannot produce its full adaptive effect.

The fourth principle: sleep is the primary anabolic window. The growth hormone pulse that supports much of the body's tissue repair occurs during slow-wave sleep. Every hour of restorative sleep is an hour of rebuilding. Every night of fragmented, unrestored sleep is a night of missed adaptation. This is why circadian restoration precedes structural rebuilding in the hierarchy.

The fifth principle: track recovery, not performance. The same measure that mattered in Chapter 8 matters here. Morning heart rate. Next-day energy. Sleep quality following sessions. If the recovery observations are consistently positive—if sessions are followed by normal fatigue that resolves overnight, by energy that is equivalent or better the next day—the load is within the adaptive window. If they are consistently negative, reduce the load before increasing it.

And finally: trust the trend. A week that felt difficult is not evidence of regression. A month that showed no progress is worth examining. The body rebuilds on its own timeline, and that timeline is longer than most people expect after years of physiologic disruption. What matters is the direction over time—not any single session, any single week, or any single comparison to your previous level of capacity.

I saw Nadia again eighteen months after our first appointment. She had returned to clinical work two days a week. Not the full-time, physically demanding work of her pre-illness career—but real clinical work, with real patients, requiring the strength and sustained physical function she had spent four years losing and one year rebuilding.

She described something that had surprised her more than the physical recovery itself. She had expected to feel relieved when the strength came back. She had not expected to feel trust. The trust that comes from movement feeling safe again. From lifting something without calculating what it would cost. From finishing a day at work and knowing, not hoping, that she would recover from it.

"The rebuilding I expected," she said. "But I didn't expect to trust it again. I had forgotten what that felt like."

In the three chapters that follow, we turn to the other side of recovery—not the restoration of function, but its protection. How to recognize regression before it becomes a setback. How to maintain what has been built. And finally, what it looks like to live in a body that has healed in order.

CHAPTER TEN

When Things Go Backwards

"Regression is not failure.
It is the system communicating that a layer
which appeared stable was not yet stable enough
to hold what was built on top of it.
The correct response is not despair.
It is precision."
—Marcus Ettinger, DC

The Week It Stopped Working

Her name is Amber. She was forty-four years old.

She had been working through the recovery sequence for seven months. As she walked into my office, I noticed something had changed in how she carried herself.

She had started to believe the recovery was real.

Six weeks earlier, she had increased her work hours. A month earlier, she had agreed to host her sister's birthday dinner, and two weeks earlier, she had told her partner she wanted to plan a trip this coming spring. These were the small commitments of a person who had begun to assume the body would cooperate because it had cooperated, consistently, for long enough that the assumption no longer felt presumptuous.

Then, on a Sunday morning in late October, she woke up at four. Not from anything in particular. She just woke and could not return to sleep. She lay in the dark listening to the familiar quality of her own mind running.

She told me later that she knew, in that moment, before the second sleepless night or the first digestive reaction or the slow return of the afternoon fatigue, what was happening. There was no evidence yet. It was just one ordinary bad night that any healthy person might have. But she knew.

"I knew it couldn't last," she said. "I had been waiting for this. I just didn't know I was waiting for it until it came."

Under the circumstances, these thoughts are understandable. They are also based on interpretation and deserve clarification. Because what Amber recognized in that moment is the first and most consequential event of regression. It is not the symptom return. It is the meaning the patient assigns to it before the evidence requires that meaning.

Over the next three weeks, the changes continued—a gradual drift. Sleep grew lighter, digestion produced occasional reactions, and her morning energy, which had been reliably present for six weeks, became inconsistent. By the third week, she was having days that felt disturbingly familiar.

But the meaning had been there from the first night.

By the time she sat across from me, she was no longer sure what to believe. Maybe she had been wrong. Maybe she had mistaken temporary improvement for recovery. Maybe the drift was not a setback at all, but a reminder of what had been true from the beginning.

"I don't know if any of it was real."

The plans had not disappeared. They had become uncertain.

Amber had stopped calculating the cost of ordinary life. And the calculation had returned, in the dark, the moment she woke at four.

The progress was real. The recovery that had occurred across those months was genuine. What had changed was not its reality; it was the set of conditions the progress depended on, and those had quietly shifted beneath it.

The building was not an illusion. The foundation had moved.

Regression Is Not a Return to the Beginning

The most important thing to understand about regression is that it is almost never a return to where you started.

A system that regresses from a more recovered state follows a different course than one that was never worked on. The regulatory foundations that were rebuilt across the recovery process do not simply disappear when the system is stressed. The nervous system that learned to tolerate more inputs before reacting does not instantly return to full reactivity. The gut that stabilized its barrier integrity does not immediately become as permeable as it was during the acute phase of illness. These changes are more durable than they feel in the middle of a regression. The body retains physiologic memory of the more recovered state, and it returns to it more quickly than it did the first time.

What regression actually is—in most cases—is a return to the layer where stabilization was incomplete. It is the specific layer that was not yet fully consolidated when the load above it was placed on it. Not the beginning of the hierarchy. The affected layer is often one or two levels below where the person currently is, not four or five.

Regression is not a return to the beginning. It is a communication from a system that has been asked to hold more than it currently can. The appropriate response is to reduce the load—not to abandon the work.

The calculation returns during regression, but it asks a different question. It no longer asks whether recovery was real, only what the body needs right now.

This does not make regression easy. The physiologic and emotional difficulties are real, and neither should be minimized. But the interpretation of regression as evidence that the recovery was false—that the body cannot sustain healing, that the progress was borrowed rather than built—is almost never accurate, and acting on that interpretation produces exactly the wrong response.

What It Feels Like: Three Patterns of Backward Movement

Not all regression feels the same. And because it does not feel the same, it does not require the same response. Understanding which pattern is operating is the first step toward responding appropriately rather than reactively.

The first pattern is drift. It is the earliest and subtlest form of backward movement, and the one most frequently missed. Drift is the regression that comes with a built-in alibi. A stretch of lighter sleep is blamed on a stressful week. An afternoon of low energy is attributed to a late lunch. A small reaction to a familiar food is explained away by a project deadline. Every signal arrives with a plausible explanation, and so each is usually dismissed rather than tracked.

Nothing is terrible. But something has narrowed.

What makes drift difficult is that every individual change feels too small to matter. The person notices it, dismisses it, notices it again, dismisses it again, and often does not recognize the pattern until it has been present for weeks.

The system is still functional. Its margin has thinned.

Drift is not a crisis. It is a signal. The recovery is not failing—the system is communicating that it is being asked to carry more than it currently can. The correct response is not alarm. It is attention. Patients who have learned to recognize drift can intercept it at this level—before it develops into something more significant—with relatively modest adjustments.

Often, the correct response is simply to reduce demand slightly, reinforce the routines that were supporting recovery, and watch closely to see whether the system returns to its previous margin.

The second pattern is layer regression. This is when the symptoms that characterized a specific earlier phase of the recovery begin to return in a recognizable way. The food reactivity pattern that was characteristic of the immune stabilization phase. The morning activation failure and evening wiring that characterized the circadian repair phase. The post-exertional crash that characterized the energy recovery phase. Something specific and recognizable has come back, and it is no longer a general sense of difficulty. It is a named experience returning.

There is something strange about layer regression that patients often describe: the symptoms are familiar in a way that is simultaneously alarming and oddly grounding. The body is producing a familiar signal from a known layer, and those signals have known responses.

Layer regression is more significant than drift, but it is still interpretable. It tells you something specific: the regulatory function of a particular layer has been sufficiently stressed to produce its characteristic symptoms again. The response is a deliberate return to the foundational practices of that layer, reduced demand on the layers above it, and enough time for stability to return. The system has been through this before, and it returns more quickly than it arrived the first time.

The third pattern is foundation regression. This is the most significant form of backward movement—and fortunately the rarest in a system that has genuinely worked through the recovery hierarchy. It is marked by the return of the amplification phenomenon from the earliest phase of illness: inputs that were previously tolerable become intolerable, treatments that were working begin to produce adverse effects, and the system's overall regulatory capacity contracts toward a restricted state. Everything feels harder. The cushion that had been there is gone.

Foundation regression is different from the other patterns. What makes it so discouraging is not primarily the symptom severity—though that can be significant. It is that the body stops feeling negotiable again. In drift and layer regression, the system is still responsive to relatively modest adjustments. In foundation regression, even careful inputs like the food that was safely reintroduced months ago or the supplement that had been well-tolerated can become activating. The schedule that had been holding stops holding.

The person finds themselves reconsidering decisions they had stopped reconsidering and reassessing activities that had become ordinary again. The calculation they thought they had left behind begins to return.

Foundation regression requires the approach that foundation stabilization originally required: a complete reduction in treatment complexity, a return to safety-signal interventions only, and patience with a timeline that's longer than the patient wants but shorter than the original recovery. The foundation has been built before, and the body knows the way back.

In each of these three patterns, the most important question to answer first is not "what should I add?" It is "what pattern is this?" Applying the wrong response—adding when the body needs less—can extend the regression rather than resolve it. The first task is not deciding what to do. It is understanding what the body is actually saying.

The Signals, and Why They Are Easy to Miss

Most major regressions begin long before they are recognized. The collapse, when it comes, may feel sudden, but it was not sudden. It was a process that became an event, with weeks of subtle signals accumulating until it finally demanded acknowledgment.

Although people experience regression differently, the early signals are remarkably consistent. Sleep quality is usually the first to shift. It is not a sudden return to the worst nights of the illness, but a gradual fragmentation. Slightly more waking in the second half of the night and mornings that feel a little less refreshed than they used to. Followed by a subtle energy dip that had been absent.

Gut-related reactivity often follows. A food that had been successfully reintroduced months earlier—one of the small victories of the recovery—begins to produce occasional mild reactions, and the digestive consistency that had been improving begins to vary. Activity recovery begins to narrow. The run that used to be unremarkable leaves the body slightly more tired the next morning.

And there is often a quality of physiologic background noise—not pain, not anxiety, but a slightly elevated baseline activation that makes rest feel less restful and effort feel more effortful.

Part of what makes these signals easy to miss is that none of them is especially meaningful on its own. A poor night, a tired day, a mild reaction—each is part of ordinary life. The body rarely communicates impending regression through a single dramatic event. It communicates through patterns, and patterns take time to become visible.

Here is where the difficulty lies. Every signal presents the same decision: whether to track it or explain it away. It rarely feels like a decision. Some people assign meaning too early, mistaking a single bad night for the beginning of a regression. Most do the opposite. They accumulate weeks of evidence before allowing themselves to recognize the pattern.

The impulse to explain it away is not an irrational assessment. It is a form of self-protection.

Recognizing drift signals requires admitting something that many recovering patients are deeply reluctant to admit: that things are not as stable as they appeared. This is not merely a physiologic observation. For someone who has told their family things are improving, who has perhaps begun to identify as a person who is getting better rather than a person who is managing illness—acknowledging the signals means confronting the possibility that the story they have been building might need revision. That is not a small thing. People resist it, often unconsciously, by finding alternative explanations for each signal individually, and never allowing the pattern to cohere into something that requires a response.

The internal monologue of that postponement is recognizable to almost everyone who has been through a regression. It's just stress. It's just a bad week. I'm still better than I was six months ago. I probably overdid it on Saturday. Things will settle once this project ends. Each is often partly true. Each is also a way of explaining the signal away.

This is why the moment of early recognition so often passes without action.

When a regression pattern begins, the signals often appear before their meaning becomes clear. The difficulty is not in seeing them. It is in permitting that meaning—before the pattern accumulates past the point where a modest intervention can resolve it.

Why the Foundation Moves

The recovery hierarchy is not a staircase that locks behind you as you climb it. It is more like a building whose lower floors have been strengthened and can support far more weight than they once could. Those improvements do not disappear when the structure is stressed. But under sufficient sustained load, strain usually appears first at the level where stabilization remains least complete.

The nervous system foundation, once recalibrated, is still susceptible to extraordinary demand. It will hold its new setting under ordinary conditions. But extraordinary conditions—a significant illness, a prolonged period of severe stress, a major life disruption, extended sleep deprivation—can recalibrate it back toward the sensitized state. Not necessarily to the starting point, but downward from where it had reached.

The same principle applies throughout the hierarchy. Recovery creates greater stability. It does not create permanent immunity to future load.

The most common trigger for this movement is not usually a single dramatic event, though it can be—an acute viral illness, for example. More often, it comes from accumulated demand. Recovery does not occur in a protected environment, as life continues during the healing process and continues after it. A period of sustained professional pressure. A difficult relationship situation that generates weeks of background stress. An illness in the family that simultaneously disrupts sleep schedules and meal timing.

None of these events felt like a crisis while they were happening, and that is what makes the pattern so difficult to recognize. The cost is paid gradually, and the system often does not present the bill until weeks later.

These are not failures. They are the ordinary contingencies of a life, and a fully recovered system would absorb them without incident. A system that has recently completed the recovery sequence—whose regulatory margins, while restored, are not yet as wide as those of a system that was never disrupted—may find that sustained accumulated demand exceeds its current capacity. Not because the recovery was false. Because recovery builds resilience; it does not eliminate limits.

Understanding this changes the meaning of regression entirely. The recovery was real. The progress was real. Regression is not the loss of those gains. It is the body's response to a period in which accumulated demand exceeded its current capacity. The system is not communicating failure. It is communicating that the load became too great for too long.

The Counter-Intuitive Response

This is where most people get it wrong.

It's rarely in understanding the framework. Most patients grasp the concept of regression fairly quickly once it's explained. Where they struggle is in the response. The correct way to handle regression runs counter to our natural instinct and to many of the strategies commonly recommended in chronic illness care. It takes real conviction to follow it.

The instinct, when symptoms return, is to escalate. To do more. Reintroduce something that was previously helpful. Push harder at the practices that had been working. Tighten the diet again. Start monitoring more closely. Look for the next intervention.

The logic feels sound. Things were going in the right direction. Now they are not. Something must have stopped working. Something new must be needed.

The logic, though, has a flaw in the context of regulatory regression. Following it—escalating when the correct response is to reduce—is one of the most reliable ways to turn a manageable drift into a significant setback.

Regression in this context is a load failure, not a treatment failure. The system has more demand on it than its current regulatory capacity can manage. Adding intervention—which is a physiologic demand on a system with a regulatory budget—adds to a load that is already excessive. Even if the intervention is perfectly chosen, even if it directly addresses the layer that has regressed, it cannot help a system that is too loaded to process the help. The timing problem that governs the entire recovery sequence does not suspend during regression. It intensifies.

The correct response is to reduce and return to the last point of stability.

Pause the most recently introduced treatment. Reduce the physical demand. Simplify the dietary approach. Reinforce the schedule. Return to the practices that restored stability before.

Give the system the physiologic space to restabilize at the current layer before asking anything more of it.

This mistake is especially common in the patients most invested in their recovery: the disciplined patient who over-responds. This is the person who built a rigorous protocol and learned that consistency, effort, and careful attention to inputs produced the recovery they achieved. When regression appears, they reach for those same tools. More structure. More restriction. More tracking. More intervention. More discipline. Each of these responses is the calculation in motion—searching for something to solve, something to add, something the body might require.

The behavior is understandable. The very habits that built the recovery can become the habits that prolong the regression.

The body in this state needs reduced load, predictability, and time, even when urgency, activation, and pressure make immediate action feel like the correct move. The body is asking for quiet. The person is generating noise. And the noise—the physiologic activation of urgency, the cortisol of fear, the autonomic cost of trying to force a quick resolution—is a form of demand on a system that is already past its capacity.

The system needs the conditions under which its own regulatory capacity can recover—which are almost always conditions of lower demand, not higher. The effort that built the recovery is different from the effort that restores after regression.

When the system is overloaded, the answer is always less. Less demand, less input, less complexity. Until the regulatory capacity has been restored to the point where the system can accept more again. Adding to an overloaded system does not accelerate recovery. It extends regression.

What to Do

The practical response to regression follows a principle that appears throughout this book: the correct intervention is aimed at the earliest layer of instability, not at the most visible symptom.

The first step is identifying which pattern is operating. Is this drift? Layer regression? Foundation regression? The answer determines the scale of the response. Drift requires modest adjustment. Layer regression requires a more deliberate return to the practices of the affected layer. Foundation regression requires a return to the earliest stabilization work. Applying a foundation regression response to drift produces over-treatment. Applying a drift response to foundation regression produces under-treatment. The pattern identification comes first.

The second step is to reduce demand. Not to stop everything and not to abandon the recovery. But to recognize that the system is communicating a capacity limit and to respect that limit rather than push through it. For most patients, this means a temporary reduction in physical activity, in complexity, and in the number of inputs being managed simultaneously. It also means returning to the foundational practices that support the earliest layer of the hierarchy: consistent sleep timing, consistent meals, the breathing practice, and the daily nature exposure that the autonomic system uses as its primary safety signal.

The third step is time, and it takes as long as is required. This is the part that is most difficult for the patients who are most committed to recovery and who understandably want to do something active in response to the setback. It is a period of reduced demand and increased consistency, during which the layer that has destabilized has the conditions and time it needs to restabilize.

The patients who return to stability the quickest are almost never the ones who pressed hardest in the regression window. They are the ones who reduced demand, waited, and let the system demonstrate its own capacity to return.

Amber did this work. It took three weeks—not three months, not a restart from the beginning. Three weeks of reduced demand, restored fundamentals, and time. At the end of those three weeks, the sleep had returned to where it had been. The digestive stability had returned. And the morning energy had returned.

But something else had returned too, and she described it in a way I have not forgotten. She said she felt less afraid of going backwards. Because she had gone backwards and now knew how to recognize it, what it required, and that it was finite. The regression had been frightening primarily because it was unfamiliar territory. It was less frightening the second time, because she understood it.

Two weeks after stability returned, she made plans for the weekend away she had deferred during the regression. She made the plans, and she did not build an exit into them.

The regression had not removed the trust she had begun to develop. If anything, surviving it had strengthened it.

The calculation had not disappeared completely. But it was no longer making the decisions.

The System That Regresses Is Not the System That Started

Underneath nearly every regression is the same fear: "I don't know if any of it was real."

The system that regresses is not the system that entered recovery. That system was trying to function without sufficient regulatory reserve. This one has already rebuilt much of it. The regression reflects a temporary mismatch between capacity and demand, not a loss of everything that was built.

The clearest expression of this is what happens to the fear. The first regression in a system that has been working through recovery is almost always the most frightening—not because it is the most severe, but because it is the most uncertain. The person does not know whether the recovery was real. They do not know how far back they will go. They do not know whether what happened before can happen again. All of that uncertainty and self-doubt amplifies the physiologic experience of the regression itself.

The second regression, in a person who has navigated the first, is experienced differently. Not comfortably. But with more orientation. The person knows this territory. They have now seen it from both sides, and they have evidence, not just belief, that the body can return. That evidence does not eliminate the difficulty. But it fundamentally changes its meaning.

That understanding—the recognition of regression as physiologic communication rather than physiologic betrayal—is one of the most durable things a person can carry into the later stages of recovery.

Recovery that has endured regression builds experience, and experience is more enduring than hope.

Foundation Work You Can Do Now

The practice for this chapter is not to do more. It is to recognize the pattern before it becomes undeniable.

Begin tracking five markers consistently: energy, digestion, sleep quality, stress tolerance, and recovery from any physical activity. Not obsessively and not in a way that may generate anxiety about each fluctuation. Do this once or twice weekly. Enough to know your baseline and notice when something has shifted from it across consecutive days rather than a single one.

The purpose of keeping this log is to identify trends, not one good day here or one bad day there. A single day of lighter sleep is not a signal. Four consecutive days of lighter or less restorative sleep is a trend. Reduced stress tolerance or slower recovery from activity is a pattern worth logging. The log makes the pattern visible. And seeing the pattern early—before the drift has become layer regression, before layer regression has become foundation regression—is what keeps the response proportionate.

When several markers have remained below your established baseline long enough to reveal a pattern, that is the moment to respond. To return to the foundational practices, reduce any recently added inputs, and give the system time. Do not escalate or add.

When the instinct says to do something, the response should be to do less.

The response should be calmer than the instinct.

For most people, the difficulty is not the tracking. Keeping a log is straightforward. The harder skill—and the one the chapter has been building toward—is what you do with what the log shows. Many people already sense the drift before the data confirms it. They feel it in the slightly less restorative sleep, the slightly heavier quality of their days, the slightly narrower margin before something feels like too much. The log's power lies in its simplicity. It externalizes the drift and makes it harder to explain away.

The log can only show you the pattern. It cannot make you willing to respond before the system forces you to. The body already knows how to move toward stability. Your role is to recognize when it needs the conditions that allow it to do so. That willingness—to respond early, to reduce demand before the drift becomes layer regression, to trust that a smaller correction now prevents a larger one later—is the real skill this chapter is trying to develop. Not better monitoring. Earlier recalibration. Those are not the same thing.

Backward movement is not lost recovery. It is the body communicating that the current load has exceeded the current capacity. When that message is recognized early and the response is proportionate, the system almost always finds its way back to stability.

CHAPTER ELEVEN

What Staying Well Actually Requires

"Long-term stability depends less on eliminating stress and more on maintaining proportionality between physiologic demand and recovery capacity. That proportionality, once understood, can be actively preserved. And actively preserving it is what staying well looks like."
—Marcus Ettinger, DC

The Question Everyone Asks

At some point during a successful recovery, a question emerges. And that question can tell me more about where a person is in the process than almost anything else.

The question is: how long do I have to keep doing this?

It's a reasonable question and deserves an honest answer.

The honest answer has two parts.

The first part: the foundational practices—the consistent wake time, the morning light, the meal rhythm, the breathing, the daily movement, and the evening routine—are not a treatment protocol. They describe how a body that wants to stay healthy needs to interface with the world. They are not temporary interventions that can be stopped once recovery is established. They are the conditions under which recovery is sustained and health is maintained. And for most people who have experienced significant chronic illness, the conditions that contributed to the illness in the first place—the schedule irregularity, the light environment, the chronic stress, the accumulated physiologic burden—are still present in some form in the world they are returning to.

The practices are not the treatment. They are the biologic signals that stability is built on.

The second part: the specific clinical interventions—the supplements, the targeted protocols, the regular monitoring—do have an endpoint. The goal of every clinical intervention in the EFP framework is to restore the body's ability to regulate itself so that the intervention is no longer needed, or is needed less often. The goal is not indefinite management. There is a meaningful difference between a body that requires continuous external support to maintain its function and one that has regained the ability to maintain that function on its own. The latter is the goal. It is achievable. And recognizing when it has been achieved—and adjusting accordingly—is one of the most important clinical judgments in the entire process.

But beneath this question is often another one that patients are not asking directly, yet is just as important. It is a question about trust: Can my body continue without external input?

This fear is logical. The person who has spent months or years in careful recovery has learned to rely on structure. The consistent schedule. The supplement protocol. The monitoring habits. The deliberate pacing. These were not merely helpful. They were the scaffolding on which the recovery was built. And as the moment approaches to remove some of that scaffolding, doubt can creep in: what if it was the scaffolding holding everything up, and not the structure beneath it?

"What if I stop and it all comes back?" I hear this doubt more often than I would like. Sometimes in those exact words. Sometimes in the more general form of reluctance to reduce anything—a hesitation to stop the supplement, lower the dose, or let go of the careful management that has felt like protection for so long.

The person trusts the protocol. They are not yet sure they trust the body.

Doubt is not a failure of the recovery process. For some, it is a natural part of the process. Because the protocol was always working toward one outcome: a body that no longer needs the protocol. And the only way to discover whether that outcome has been reached is to extend the same careful attention to the transition out of treatment that was given to the recovery itself. We reduce support purposefully and objectively, watching what the body demonstrates rather than assuming that the support must continue forever or that it can all be removed at once.

The Difference Between Treatment and Maintenance

Treatment and maintenance are not the same thing. They are two different ways of working with the body—each with its own purpose, its own definition of success, and its own relationship to the hierarchy we have been building throughout this book.

Treatment is what we have been doing in the preceding chapters: identifying the layer of the hierarchy that is most compromised, providing the specific interventions needed to help it stabilize, and maintaining that stability long enough for the layer above it to become accessible. Treatment is targeted. It can be intensive or supportive in nature. In either case, it is directed toward a specific deficit and continues until the body can reliably maintain that function on its own.

Maintenance is something different. It is not merely the absence of treatment. It is the active preservation of the conditions that allow the body to keep organizing itself.

The goal of maintenance is to preserve the stability that has been achieved. It is the ongoing work of keeping demand and recovery in balance so that health can sustain itself without the intensive support that treatment once required.

Treatment builds. Maintenance protects.

This distinction—between correcting a deficit and sustaining a balance—is crucial to understanding what maintenance involves. Because the most common mistake in the maintenance phase is the opposite of neglect. Patients carry the intensity and vigilance of active treatment into a period that no longer requires it.

Patients who have been through a demanding recovery process learn to monitor symptoms carefully and respond quickly to changes. They keep their protocol rigorous and their schedule defended. They sometimes find it difficult to release that vigilance even when the system no longer needs it. The hyperawareness that was appropriate during recovery becomes a habit the body no longer requires. The careful assessment before every commitment. The scanning after every meal. The mental calculation of energy reserves before saying yes to anything.

These self-preservation habits were not irrational then. They were the correct response to a body that was still unreliable. But they persist, in many people, past the point where the body has become reliable again.

A body that is managed beyond what it needs receives a message: something still requires management, and the system is not yet ready to be trusted on its own. Repeated consistently, that message is not neutral. The body continues receiving the impression that it remains fragile, and it keeps the person from becoming as well as they could be because of the ongoing physiologic cost of the sustained vigilance.

Maintenance requires a different relationship with the body—one that shifts the focus from treating the body as something that might fail at any moment to treating it as something that has demonstrated it knows how to function.

What the Body Needs to Stay Well

The maintenance requirements of a recovered body are considerably less demanding than the recovery requirements of an ill one. Patients sometimes arrive at the maintenance phase having absorbed the intensity of the recovery process and assume that maintenance will require the same level of intensity, sometimes indefinitely. It does not. It needs reinforcement.

Treatment corrects the deficit, and reinforcement helps preserve the function that has been restored. These are different clinical tasks. A body in the maintenance phase has already rebuilt many of the capacities that were compromised during illness—a nervous system that can regulate itself more reliably, an immune system that is less reactive, a circadian rhythm that has regained its stability, and an energy-production system that can adapt to ordinary life without becoming overwhelmed. What it requires now is periodic support for what has already been restored.

The nervous system that has been recalibrated from a sensitized state to a regulated one does not require daily interventions to stay regulated—it requires the absence of the conditions that originally sensitized it, and the continued presence of the safety signals that supported its recalibration. The morning light. The consistent schedule. The daily movement. The breathing practice from Chapter 3 maintained at a frequency that keeps the nervous system supported—not at the intensity required during recovery, but at a consistent level of practice that keeps the nervous system in the habit of regulation.

The immune system that has been stabilized does not require ongoing gut protocols and barrier support indefinitely. It requires the continued absence of the dietary chaos and schedule irregularity that were degrading it. There will also be periods when physiologic demands increase. Those periods are often highly individual: an acute illness, sustained stress, a major life disruption, caring for a newborn, or traveling abroad. During those times, temporary reinforcement may be appropriate until ordinary maintenance is sufficient again.

The circadian clock that has been entrained does not require perfect adherence to every timing signal every day of the rest of a person's life. Holding the anchors approximately eighty percent of the time is usually sufficient—enough regularity that the clock can absorb occasional disruption without losing its entrainment.

The mitochondria that have restored reliable energy production do not require full recovery protocols after every modest demand. What they require is proportionality—demand followed by recovery, activity followed by physiologic completion rather than ongoing strain, and enough rhythm in daily life that the body continues to interpret ordinary activity as manageable rather than threatening.

The distinction that matters is between a body that maintains itself with occasional reinforcement and one that is maintained by continuous external intervention. The first is what recovery makes possible. The second is what chronic illness imposed. The goal of the entire preceding sequence has been to restore the body's own regulatory authority—to return to it the capacity to manage its own systems without requiring constant external support.

Maintenance means preserving recovered regulation—not continuously compensating for failed regulation. Its work is to create the conditions under which that regulation continues.

The Proportionality Principle

One of the most useful concepts for understanding what long-term health maintenance requires is what I call the proportionality principle. It's more useful than any specific intervention or supplement protocol, and once you have it, it simplifies the maintenance question considerably.

The principle is this: long-term stability of one's health depends on maintaining proportionality between physiologic demand and recovery capacity. The practical expression of this principle is simple: reducing unnecessary demand where possible and building enough recovery capacity to absorb the demands that remain.

The world will always possess the potential to generate stress. Illness, loss, professional pressure, relationship difficulty, financial strain, or the accumulated demands of ordinary life—these are problems we all face; they are features of the human experience. It is wishful thinking to believe a recovery protocol requires eliminating them, or could do so even if it tried. What a recovery protocol can manage—what the hierarchy we have built throughout this book is specifically designed to support—is the relationship between demand and capacity. When demand and capacity are proportionate, the system can absorb the demand, recover from it, and return to baseline. When demand chronically exceeds capacity—when the life being lived is always asking more of the system than the system can absorb and recover from—the system drifts. We described this drift toward a dysregulated state in Chapter 10.

We can't eliminate demand, but we can expand capacity. We can't make stress disappear, but we can ensure that the recovery infrastructure is sufficient to manage it when it inevitably arrives. We can't protect ourselves from living. But we can build a body that can fully participate in life without requiring constant protection.

What trusting proportionality actually feels like, for someone who has lived for years in the calculated management of a dysregulated system, is hard to describe unless you've lived in it. It feels like permission. Permission to say yes to things without first running the energy calculation. Permission to make plans without building in the recovery buffer. Permission to be present in a situation without monitoring what the body is doing in the background. The person who has internalized proportionality does not stop being aware of their body; they just stop being governed by it. There is an enormous difference between those two things.

This is a different relationship to health than most people with a history of chronic illness have ever had. It is not the vigilant avoidance of triggers or the careful management of exposure. It is the confident management of capacity: a body that trusts itself and a person who trusts their body.

It begins with increasing demand deliberately. Allowing recovery to complete before adding more. Accepting the occasional demanding week without assuming that every challenge requires retreat. And responding early when life begins asking more of the body than it can comfortably recover from.

Health is not fragility protected from life. It is capacity that can absorb life.

Reading the Early Signals

The maintenance phase introduces a specific and important challenge that does not exist during recovery: the temptation to ignore the early signals of drift because life has finally become something worth living and is now actively being lived.

During the recovery process, monitoring the body's signals was not difficult because motivation to be well was the driver. In the maintenance phase, this changes. The person is well, or well enough. Well enough that ordinary life has become accessible again. The forward orientation has returned, and the careful calculation before every commitment has started to feel less necessary. And it is precisely at this moment that the early signals of drift become easiest to miss.

Health creates possibility. Possibility creates demand. As life expands, so do the demands placed upon the system.

The catch is that demand can increase gradually enough that the imbalance is easy to miss. When recovery capacity does not expand with it, strain accumulates quietly and often becomes visible only after it has been present for some time.

The pattern is recognizable. The person starts saying yes again. A dinner they would have declined six months ago. A work project they would have managed more slowly. A social commitment they would have spaced out more deliberately. Each yes is an earned yes. It feels like evidence of recovery—proof that the life they worked toward has become available to them. And it is, until it is slightly too much, or too often, and the first drift signals appear.

Here is what makes this moment difficult: the person does not want to see the signals. They have just begun to stop organizing their life around illness, and acknowledging that something is shifting feels like going backward. In the brief window between feeling well enough to resume ordinary life and exceeding proportionality without realizing it, the early signals pass unaddressed. Not because the person missed them. Because they recognized them and chose, understandably, not to take them seriously yet.

The early signals of drift are the same ones described in Chapter 10. What changes in the maintenance phase is the context in which they appear. The person now has strong motivation to explain them away. It's a busy month. I'm adjusting. Things will settle. Each of these can be true. The distinction between normal variation and genuine drift is the same one Chapter 10 described—a sustained pattern rather than an isolated bad day. The practice of maintenance is not about constant monitoring; it is proportional response. It is the willingness, when the pattern becomes obvious, to respond to what it is showing rather than to the story about why it doesn't mean anything yet.

Learning to Stop Monitoring

There is a transition that happens somewhere in the maintenance phase that may be hard for some to recognize—it is the transition from living like a sick person to living like a well one.

The person who has been seriously ill for a significant period of time, as I've mentioned earlier, develops a specific relationship with their own body, one organized around monitoring, calculation, and management. Before agreeing to plans, trying a new food, or committing to an activity, they assess and consider the potential costs or outcomes. Do I have the energy? Is the food safe? Will I be able to recover from this before the next thing? This is not neurosis. This is the intelligent, learned response of someone whose body was genuinely unreliable and who had no choice but to build a system to manage that unpredictability. At the time, it was the correct response to the situation.

There comes a point, though, where the situation changes, and the body becomes reliable.

The habits that were correct responses to an unreliable body persist into the maintenance phase, sometimes for months, sometimes longer. Letting them go requires trusting something that was not trustworthy for a long time. The calculation became the default response, and the monitoring continued out of habit. Over time, the monitoring stops feeling like something they do and starts feeling like who they are. Where the habit persists, releasing it is part of the maintenance phase.

What the maintenance phase ultimately requires, at its deepest level, is learning to stop doing some of this. Not all at once, but deliberately—extending the range of life lived without physiologic negotiation, one increment at a time, until the default relationship with the body is participation rather than management.

In real life, this looks like making a plan without first calculating whether the energy budget will support it. Agreeing to something spontaneously, without the pre-assessment. Eating at a restaurant without reviewing the menu for potential reactions. Traveling without building in the extra recovery day. It means simply living—and discovering that the body, having healed in order, moves through ordinary life without requiring the constant oversight that illness made necessary.

The first time a person notices that they have not once checked in on how their body is doing—it can feel strange. The monitoring was so habitual that its absence is noticeable.

The body becomes a given again rather than a variable.

One patient described noticing, midway through a conversation with a friend she had not seen in months, that she had been fully present for the entire lunch—not once tracking what the meal was costing her or calculating whether she had enough left for the evening. She had simply been there, enjoying the meal and the friendship. Ordinary had never felt so good.

That transition—from a calculated life to an uncalculated life—is not the absence of self-awareness. It is the restoration of normal self-awareness, the kind that does not require constant active engagement to maintain. The person who has completed this transition is no longer managing the body as an adversary. They are living with it as something reliable again.

What Changes and What Does Not

Patients sometimes ask me, as they approach the end of active treatment, whether they will always be more vulnerable than someone who has never been significantly ill.

I answer this question acknowledging two things simultaneously.

The first is that a significant period of chronic illness often leaves a lasting imprint on physiology. A shift in the way the system operates, which means the recovered person is not quite the same as the person who was never ill.

This does not mean the body is fragile. It means the margin for sustained imbalance is often a bit narrower. Most people who recover return to a normal level of function. They may, however, need to be somewhat more deliberate and diligent about the maintenance principles we have discussed in this chapter: keeping a consistent schedule, allowing recovery after periods of elevated demand, and responding to early signals before they become larger problems. This is where a little post-illness effort can pay enormous dividends over the course of a lifetime.

This is not a reason for despair. It is simply a reason to remain in a relationship with the body that was rebuilt. And the word remain is important because the difference between the recovered person and someone without the same history is not the difference between illness and health.

The second thing I acknowledge is this: a history of illness does not have to permanently diminish the body's capacity to adapt. In many cases, it can actually sharpen it in important ways.

The person who has been through significant chronic illness and recovered has done something that a person who has never had to navigate serious illness has never been required to do. They have learned to read their body's signals with a precision most people never develop. They respond to those signals early and proportionally, and they distinguish between the normal noise of daily variation and the clearer signal of genuine drift.

That knowledge is a hard-earned intelligence—one that most people never have reason to cultivate.

Many of the patients I have worked with who have recovered from chronic illness describe their relationship with their own physiology, post-recovery, as better than it was before the illness began. Why? They have put in the time and effort through recovery and into maintenance. They understand what their body requires because they can now interpret what it is communicating and respond early enough to prevent the accumulation of unresolved demand that contributed to the original illness. That knowledge, invaluable and earned through enormous difficulty, does not disappear when the illness does. It becomes the foundation of a different kind of health—not random good health, but earned and deserved health.

The Long Game

There is a phrase I use with patients approaching the transition from active treatment to maintenance. It captures what the maintenance phase actually requires.

The phrase is simple: play the long game.

Not in the sense of delayed gratification or sustained effort toward a distant goal. In the more specific sense of making decisions—about how much to commit to, how hard to push, how quickly to add new demands—with the knowledge that the hierarchy has a long memory and a reliable logic, and that the decisions made in any given week are not just affecting that week. They are affecting the regulatory state of a system that will respond to those decisions in the weeks and months that follow.

The person playing the long game thinks differently about time. The crisis-response mode of active illness asks one question: how do I get through this week? The stewardship mode of maintained health asks a different one: what am I building across this month, this season, and this year? The person who is getting through the week is reacting. The person playing the long game is tending. These are fundamentally different relationships with time and with the body.

Playing the long game means choosing the full recovery after a demanding session, not the truncated one that saves time today at the cost of tomorrow. It means keeping the wake time on the weekend when sleeping in would feel better, because the clock's anchor matters more than the single morning. It means reducing the load when drift signals appear, before the drift becomes regression—even when the reduction feels like unnecessary caution because nothing has fully broken yet. It means understanding that the body is not a machine that can be pushed hard and then serviced. It is a living system with regulatory dynamics that extend across days and weeks and months, and that responds to the pattern of how it is treated, not just to any single day.

It's more about being intelligent than cautious. The person playing the long game understands that every meaningful decision has a trajectory—that each choice has consequences that extend beyond today. They are helping the body remain capable of fully participating in life. The advantage compounds because today's decisions become tomorrow's baseline, and with time the margin widens. A body that is consistently supported rather than consistently stressed develops increasing resilience—a widening of the adaptive window that makes ordinary life progressively less effortful and extraordinary demands progressively easier to recover from.

The patients I have worked with genuinely thrive in maintenance. Universally, they are people who have internalized the long game and have shifted from the crisis-response mode of active illness to the stewardship mode of sustained health. They also understand that the hierarchy is not something you build once and walk away from. It is something you live within and maintain.

It is the practice of a life that works.

The Return of Ordinary Life

At some point in the maintenance phase, the final goal of the entire recovery sequence becomes visible as a lived experience.

What recovery is ultimately for is not symptom reduction, improved lab values, or a more sophisticated relationship with the body's physiology. It is the return to ordinary life without the threat of negative physiologic consequences.

Ordinary life is the life most people live without ever having to think about it. You make plans, say yes to things, go to the store, cook a meal, have a conversation, or take a trip without first calculating what it will cost your body.

The goal is not optimization, peak performance, or mastery of a complex system. The goal is freedom—the freedom to participate in life without having to think about the body all the time.

A busy week followed by an ordinary weekend rather than a recovery protocol. A conversation that runs long without the next day being organized around repair.

What makes these examples important is that they are viewed as ordinary achievements, yet illness can place them completely out of reach. They were ordinary before the illness began, and they become ordinary again once recovery is complete. That said, the person who has been through the illness and the recovery knows something that the person who never lost them cannot: that these unremarkable features of a normal life are not given. They are built. They are the downstream consequence of the work described in all the preceding chapters. The sleeping that became restorative again. The schedule that became an anchor. The pacing that allowed recovery to keep up with demand. The gradual return of reliable energy. The sequenced restoration of each layer of the hierarchy. All of it moving toward this: a day that passes without the body being the primary subject of the person's attention.

This is not the absence of awareness. The person who has recovered and maintained that recovery carries forward a kind of intelligence that illness required them to develop. They understand what the body is communicating, recognize meaningful changes earlier, and know when something requires attention and when it does not.

That awareness remains. It simply no longer occupies the center of the person's life.

The work, the people, the plans, the ordinary unremarkable texture of days that are not organized around illness. That is what recovery makes possible. The maintenance work of this chapter is what keeps it possible.

Foundation Work You Can Do Now

The practice of the maintenance phase is different from the practice of recovery. In recovery, the work was targeted—identifying the layer that needed stabilization and providing the specific inputs to achieve it. In maintenance, the work is more like tending than building, and requires less precision and intensity than recovery did. The focus is on consistency, proportionality, and the willingness to respond early when the body communicates that something has shifted.

Keep the foundational anchors permanent. The consistent wake time, the morning light, the meal rhythm, the breathing practice, the daily movement—these are not interventions to be stopped when recovery is established. They are the conditions under which the recovered state remains stable. They do not require vigilance. They require consistency.

Reduce the targeted clinical interventions deliberately and gradually, in conversation with the practitioners working with you. The criterion for reduction is less about how long you have been taking something and more about whether the body continues to function well without it under the demands of ordinary life. Remove one input at a time. Observe across two to three weeks before removing another. The body will demonstrate what it continues to need and what it no longer does—if given the time and consistent conditions to do so.

Track the five early warning signals as background awareness—not the foreground monitoring of the recovery phase, but a light and consistent attentiveness to sleep quality, food tolerance, activity recovery, stress tolerance, and whether everyday life feels a little easier or a little harder than it did a week or two ago. When two or more of these shift consistently across more than a day or two, respond before the pattern becomes something that requires more than a return to basics.

And learn, gradually, to extend the range of life that happens without calculation. Not all at once. And not recklessly. But deliberately.

The body that has healed in order has earned the right to be trusted.

One patient described the moment she realized she had moved from recovery into maintenance. She noticed it on an ordinary Tuesday. Not because something significant happened, but because nothing did. She had gotten through the day—a full day of meetings, an evening walk, and a dinner she had not planned in advance—without once checking in on how her body was doing. She had just lived the day. She realized this at the end of it, getting ready for bed, and she held the thought for a moment before setting it aside. It was just a Tuesday. But it was also exactly what the work had been for.

CHAPTER TWELVE

The Whole Picture

"Chronic illness is not a mystery without a solution.
It is a hierarchy without a sequence.
Give it the sequence, and the body does the rest."
—Marcus Ettinger, DC

Claire, Without the Binder

Claire came back to see me about eighteen months after that first appointment. The one where she had arrived with the binder.

She did not have the binder with her. I noticed this before she said anything, and it struck me as the most significant clinical data point of the entire appointment.

She sat down and looked at me across the desk—the same desk, the same chair—and I could see immediately that something fundamental had changed. Not just that she felt better, though she did. Something in the way she inhabited the appointment. She was not braced for disappointment. She was not front-loading the credible details of her history in anticipation of skepticism. She was simply there—present, unguarded, carrying none of the exhaustion of a person who has spent years explaining something that resists explanation.

She told me what the previous eighteen months had looked like. The early months, working through the foundation work—the breathing, the nature exposure, the schedule anchoring—that had felt, at the time, like very little. "I kept waiting for something to happen," she said. "I kept expecting a treatment. And you kept telling me that what we were doing was the treatment."

The turning point, she said, had come about five months in. Not a dramatic change. A week in which she had not crashed. And then another week. And then a month in which she had been able to eat at a family dinner without spending the next two days recovering from it. "I almost didn't notice," she said. "That's how gradual it was. And then one day I realized I had stopped keeping track."

After years of the exhausting vigilance of chronic illness—the food diary, the symptom log, the daily assessment of how the body was doing—she had stopped keeping track. Because there was nothing that felt alarming anymore.

For someone living with chronic illness, no longer needing to keep track is rarely accidental. It usually reflects a change in how life is organized and experienced. The binder had not just been a medical record. It had been the external embodiment of a life built around threat management. Every page of it represented a decision made through the filter of illness: what could be eaten, what could be risked, what could be planned, what needed to be avoided.

And when the binder was no longer necessary, it was not just the binder that was put away. It was the way of life the binder had come to represent—the careful calculation before every commitment, the morning assessment of what the body could tolerate today, the involuntary scanning that had been so constant she had not known it had stopped until she noticed its absence.

Recovery became visible not when her symptoms disappeared, but when vigilance stopped organizing her life.

The binder was at home. In a closet, she thought. She hasn't opened it in years.

David, Two Years Later

I also heard from David about eighteen months after his own treatment had ended—not an appointment, just a brief note. He had completed a half-marathon he had always wanted to run, and he had followed up by registering for another one the following spring. These were goals that at one point he thought were unattainable. They were now a reality. But that was not the reason he wrote.

He wrote because his eldest son had come home that week on winter break and described a pattern of symptoms that David recognized immediately. The unpredictable fatigue. He wasn't recovering from training the way he should. The sense of hitting a ceiling that had not been there before.

"I knew exactly what he was describing," David wrote. "My first reaction surprised me. There was no panic. For the first time in my life, when someone I cared about described feeling that way, I had something useful to say about it. I knew what it was, I knew what it wasn't, and I knew what to do. That felt like the most important thing this whole process gave me. Not the half-marathon. That."

For the first time, he was able to offer someone else the kind of reassurance and guidance he had once needed himself.

He went on to describe something that I have thought about since. He had spent most of his adult life, he said, in what he could now recognize as an adversarial relationship with his own body. Not through anger or resentment, but through constant management. His body became something he pushed, managed, and treated as an instrument to be maintained rather than as something with its own intelligence and its own requirements. When it crashed, he assumed it was failing. When it refused to adapt to training, he assumed it was being difficult. He pushed harder. He escalated. He brought the same problem-solving energy to his physiology that had worked everywhere else in his life, and watched it not work here, without understanding why.

What the recovery process gave him was not just the return of function. It was a fundamentally different interpretation of what his body had been doing the entire time. When it crashed, it was not failing. It was communicating. When it refused to adapt, it was not being difficult. It was being accurate—accurately reporting that the conditions for adaptation were not yet in place.

The body had been right about itself all along.

He had been the one misreading the signals.

"I used to think the body was the obstacle," he wrote. "Now I understand it was the guide. It was telling me exactly what it needed. I just didn't know how to listen. I don't assume it's failing anymore. I assume it's telling me something worth understanding."

That is what healing in order gives you. Not simply a recovered body, but a different relationship with the body you live in—one organized around listening rather than overriding, cooperation rather than management, and trust in the body's own intelligence rather than impatience with it.

Elena, Fourteen Months In

Elena was the one who had said, early in our work together, that the hardest part of being chronically ill was not the symptoms. It was that nobody had the box.

Every practitioner she had seen had a piece of the picture, a part of the puzzle, a framework that partially fit—and none of them had the box that the puzzle came in, the image on the front that told you how the pieces were supposed to relate to each other. Elena had taught high school biology for twelve years. The irony was not lost on her. She had spent her career explaining how the body's systems worked to teenagers, and she could not find anyone who could explain to her what was happening in her own body in terms that made any coherent sense.

What she meant by the box, I came to understand, was not a diagnosis. She had diagnoses. She had several of them, acquired over years of appointments with each specialist looking at a different piece of the picture.

What she meant was a framework—an explanatory structure that made all the pieces fit together. Something that explained both what was wrong and why things were wrong in this particular sequence, in this particular combination, in this particular way that kept resisting the treatments that should have worked.

Living without that kind of framework changes the experience of being ill.

When symptoms are inexplicable—following no pattern that the person can understand, worsening despite correct treatment, improving for a period, and then returning without apparent cause—the experience cannot be integrated. It cannot be understood as part of a story that makes sense. It can feel random, and living without a coherent explanation is profoundly demoralizing. The person begins to question not just their body but their perception. The practitioners they trust offer contradictory explanations. The treatments they follow produce unpredictable responses. The history accumulates and refuses to cohere, and the incoherence can become another burden to carry.

Despite appearances, the body had been coherent all along. What appeared random was never random. The symptoms followed a pattern, the setbacks followed a pattern, and even the treatments that made things worse followed a pattern. The problem was that no one had yet been looking through the right framework.

That realization changes more than an explanation. It changes a person's relationship with their own body. Instead of wondering what unexpected thing it might do next, they begin to understand that every response has meaning, even when they cannot yet see it. The doubt begins to give way to clarity.

Fourteen months after we began working together, Elena sat across from me.

"I finally have the box," she said. "Everything that confused me before—the treatments that made things worse, the recovery plateaus that made no sense, every time I got better and then didn't—it all fits now. It was all the same problem, expressed in different places."

She paused.

"I think that's what I needed most," she said. "For it to finally make sense."

I have heard some version of that from more patients than I can count. Not because understanding changes what they lived through. It doesn't. What changes is that the years stop feeling random. The contradictions begin to fit together. The history becomes something that can be understood instead of something that must simply be endured.

That understanding cannot change the past. But it can change how a person carries it.

What This Book Has Been Saying

Twelve chapters in, it is worth gathering the argument into its simplest possible form.

For many patients with chronic multi-system illness—the kind that produces overlapping symptoms across digestion, immunity, sleep, energy, mood, and metabolism, that resists diagnosis, that fails to respond predictably to treatments that should work—the most useful frame is not the disease category but the regulatory hierarchy beneath it. The body's systems are arranged in a specific order, governed by a specific sequence of signaling relationships. When the upstream systems destabilize, the downstream systems follow in predictable ways. When the upstream systems are restored in the right sequence, the downstream systems follow back.

Treatment succeeds not when it targets the most visible symptom. It succeeds when it matches the level of actual regulatory failure—when it addresses the layer that is driving the problem, in the sequence that the hierarchy requires.

The treatments were not wrong. The sequence was wrong. That distinction—between a treatment failure and a timing failure—is the central insight this book has been building toward from its first page.

Every treatment that made things worse was likely introduced before the layer below it was stable enough to absorb it. Every plateau that refused to budge was likely a layer that appeared improved but had not yet reached the signaling stability required for the one above it to engage. Every crash that followed a period of progress was likely a system advanced before its foundation was ready to hold the weight.

None of this was the body failing. None of it was a personal inadequacy. None of it was the wrong treatment. It was the wrong sequence. And sequence, unlike failure, has a correction. The correction does not require new treatments. It requires applying the treatments you may already have been using in the order that the hierarchy actually requires.

Improvement is not the same as healing. A person can feel significantly better during a vacation, a season of lower stress, or a period when life simply becomes easier to carry, even though the underlying causes of their illness remain unchanged. Symptoms often improve when demands temporarily decrease. Healing is different. It is what allows those improvements to hold when life becomes demanding again.

The body does not announce recovery. It does not produce a dramatic turning point. It produces a gradual accumulation of small changes that only become visible when you stop looking for the dramatic version and start looking for the quiet one. A week without a crash. A month without keeping track. A dinner without consequences. A half-marathon. A closet with a binder in it that hasn't been opened in seven months.

The Patients in These Pages

Throughout this book, we have followed composite patients whose experiences were drawn from patterns I have observed across thousands of clinical encounters over nearly four decades. Claire with her binder. David with his ceiling. Elena with her five diagnoses and no box to put them in. James whose protocol made him the sickest he had ever been. Rachel whose nervous system treated the world like a continuous emergency. Maria who was always one thing away from not being able to. Sophie whose list of safe foods kept shrinking. Thomas who slept fine but never felt rested. Nadia who was building on sand. Amber whose foundation moved beneath her.

These are not exceptional cases. They are representative ones. The patterns they embody appear, in one form or another, in the lives of tens of millions of people who are currently living with chronic illness that has not responded fully to standard treatment.

What the stories share is not the specific diagnosis or the specific symptom pattern. What they share is the experience of a logical physiologic process being interpreted through an illogical framework. The body was responding predictably to a regulatory hierarchy under stress.

The people living in those bodies—and the practitioners treating them—were looking for the problem in the wrong layer. They were applying solutions to symptoms rather than to the regulatory failure generating them.

The result was predictable: treatments that should work but don't, improvements that don't hold, and the mistaken impression that the body itself was resisting help.

If these stories feel familiar, they are.

You are not a difficult case. Your body has been protecting itself in the only way it knows how.

The complexity was not in the body. It was in the approach.

Each composite story in this book traces a path through recovery—different in pace, different in presentation, different in how far the illness had progressed before the sequence was established. But each arrived at the same destination: a body that was no longer the organizing problem of daily life. A life that had room in it again for things that had nothing to do with being ill. They no longer felt the need to keep track of everything.

What You Have Already

If you have read this book and begun the practices in it, you have already started.

You have a consistent wake time and morning light exposure that is anchoring your circadian clock and beginning the restoration of anticipatory morning activation. You have a breathing practice that is sending direct, daily input to the foundational layer of your regulatory hierarchy. You have a daily experience of natural environment that is reducing your nervous system's ambient threat assessment. You have consistent meal timing that is supporting your gut's self-organizing cycles and allowing your immune system's tolerance mechanisms to develop predictable inputs. You have an evening practice that is supporting the melatonin signal and the evening disengagement that restorative sleep requires.

These are not extraordinary interventions. The practices themselves are ordinary. What makes them so impactful is the understanding with which they are applied—the recognition that they are not lifestyle preferences but regulatory inputs, addressing the foundational layer of the hierarchy before the layers above it are asked to stabilize. The sequence is what changes the outcome. The same practices, applied in the wrong order or without the understanding of why they work, produce ordinary results. Applied in the right order, with the understanding that the hierarchy is real and that the foundation must be established before anything above it can hold—they produce something quite different.

These practices are not a substitute for clinical care. Significant chronic illness requires a practitioner who understands the regulatory hierarchy and can guide you through its specific requirements for your specific presentation. But the practices you have now are not nothing. They are the conditions under which clinical treatment works. For many readers, beginning them—consistently, patiently, with the understanding of why they matter—will produce changes in their physiologic baseline that no other approach has been able to produce. Because no other approach has started at the right layer.

A Note to Practitioners

If you are a practitioner reading this book—a physician, a naturopath, a chiropractor, a nurse practitioner, a functional medicine clinician, a health coach—the patients in these pages are your patients.

You have sat across the desk from Claire. You have told David that his labs were normal. You have watched James get worse on a protocol you were confident in. You have done everything the evidence supported and watched a patient not improve. I was there too.

What I know about that experience—from my own years inside it, before the sequencing principle became clear—is that it produces a specific clinical disorientation. You begin to question the treatment protocols that you have been using. You question the diagnosis, though the tests support it. You question your own judgment, which, with other patients, was correct. In the cases that persist, you may even begin to wonder whether you are missing something fundamental—whether there is a dimension of this patient's presentation that you are not equipped to address. That doubt, in a conscientious practitioner, is honest. And it is also unnecessary. The problem is almost never the treatment. It is the timing. The question is almost never which therapy—it is whether the system is currently capable of receiving it.

The framework this book describes is a sequencing principle that, once integrated into clinical thinking, changes not the treatment, but when it is introduced. It is a precise tool for a specific job: helping patients with chronic illness establish the conditions their physiology requires before recovery can proceed. The treatments remain the same. The diagnosis remains the same. What changes is the assessment of whether the system is ready to receive what you are about to offer it, and the recognition that readiness follows the hierarchy rather than the symptom.

The patients who have spent months or years in your care without measurable improvement are not treatment failures. They are often sequencing failures. And the difference between those two framings—between a patient whose body has rejected treatment and a patient who was given the right treatment in the wrong order—is the difference between a practitioner who has reached the limit of what they can offer and one who has found the next step.

Healing in Order

The title of this book is both a description and an instruction.

It is a description of what the body does when given the conditions it needs: it heals, and it heals in a specific, predictable order. The nervous system first. Then the immune system. Followed by the circadian clock, the mitochondria, and the structural support network. Lastly, the sustained, coordinated function of a body that has rebuilt its capacity from the foundation upward. This order is not a clinical preference. It is a physiologic reality, written into the architecture of a regulatory hierarchy that reflects hundreds of millions of years of biological organization.

The body heals in order because biology itself is ordered.

That order is not negotiable, but it is knowable. Knowing it changes everything about what becomes possible.

It is also an instruction. Heal in order. Not in the order of the most dramatic symptom or the most appealing intervention. In biological order. The order the hierarchy requires. The order that allows each layer to do its work and prepare the ground for the layer above it.

This instruction sounds simple. It is, in clinical practice, one of the most demanding things a patient or practitioner can commit to—because it requires resisting the impulse toward the more obvious, more immediately satisfying intervention in favor of the less obvious, slower-returning but genuinely effective one. It requires patience and consistency with a process that moves at the pace of physiology rather than the pace of urgency. It requires the willingness to interpret worsening as information rather than failure, plateaus as incomplete stabilization rather than permanent ceiling, and the body's apparent resistance as protection rather than pathology.

Throughout the entire history of a person's chronic illness, the body has been protecting itself—responding with the total, coherent intelligence of a physiologic system. Every system was responding toward the same goal, each adjusting its own function in service of the body's attempt to maintain stability under difficult conditions. The treatments that made things worse were not rejected because the body was broken. They were rejected because they arrived before the layer that needed to receive them was stable enough to do so. The body was not refusing help.

The body was refusing disorder.

It was maintaining, with whatever regulatory capacity it still had, the best version of stability available to it under the conditions that were present. That is not failure. That is biology working correctly in difficult circumstances.

Understanding this—genuinely understanding it, not just intellectually accepting it but feeling its implication for everything that has happened—changes the relationship between person and body from adversarial to collaborative. The body was working toward the same outcome you were working toward: stability, recovery, the ability to absorb what life requires without paying an impossible cost.

Give the body the right conditions. Give them in the right order. Give them the time that physiology requires. And trust—with the evidence of the preceding twelve chapters and the stories of the patients in them—that the body knows how to heal. It has always known.

What healing in order provides is the sequence.

The body is not broken. It is waiting—with a patience that exceeds anything we bring to it—for the conditions that will allow it to do what it already knows how to do.

Epilogue

Claire and David and Elena—and James, Rachel, Maria, Sophie, Thomas, Nadia, and Amber—each of them arrived where they arrived by different paths, at different speeds, with different histories and different presentations. What they share is what recovery from chronic illness looks like from the inside: not dramatic, not sudden, not the moment you hoped for and then wondered if you had imagined. It is gradual. And not without its ups and downs. It is the slow accumulation of days that no longer require negotiation and the return of plans that are made without first running the calculation. The body resuming its role as a given rather than a variable.

Each of them, at some point, had a moment they did not expect. Not a milestone.

A Tuesday, a Saturday, a morning unremarkable in every way except that it passed without the body being the subject of it. They noticed it only afterward.

And then it happened again. And then it stopped being remarkable at all.

The sequence is real.

The hierarchy holds.

The body, given the right conditions in the right order, does what it was always designed to do.

Heal in order.

The binder is in a closet. She hasn't opened it in years.

Afterword

Ten Axioms for Healing in Order

—Marcus Ettinger, DC

A note on what this is: these ten principles predate this book by fifteen years. They are what I had come to believe about the body after years of research and clinical practice, and were written down long before I had any idea they would influence a book. They are offered as condensed reminders—not a summary of the argument, but a way back into it.

1. Biology Responds to Conditions, Not to Preference.

The body does not care what we wish were true, or what we have decided to believe. It responds only to what is actually reaching it. When a conviction and a physiologic requirement collide, the body does not negotiate. It reports the outcome, and we call the report a symptom. This does not mean your convictions are wrong. It means they do not exempt you.
See Chapters 1 and 3

2. Disease Emerges When Biology Must Adapt to What It Was Never Built For.

The human body is remarkably adaptive, but adaptation has a cost and a limit. When stress, poor sleep, isolation from nature, nutritional deficiency, toxins, or unresolved inflammation persist long enough, symptoms appear—not because the body is failing, but because it is still trying to survive conditions that exceed what it can compensate for indefinitely. The body is rarely defective. It is usually prevented from completing its normal work.
See Chapters 1 and 2

3. A Nervous System That Cannot Trust the Environment Cannot Invest in Repair.

The nervous system continuously interprets whether the environment is safe, and the body acts on that interpretation. A system reading danger prioritizes defense over repair. This is not a psychological event. It is a physiologic one, and it is not corrected by thinking differently. It is corrected when the conditions around the person allow the nervous system to stop bracing.

See Chapter 5

4. You Do Not Heal Yourself. You Create the Conditions in Which Healing Becomes Possible.

No supplement, medication, practitioner, or protocol heals the body. The body heals itself, when the conditions permit. What you can change—your sleep, your light, your food, your movement, your relationships, your environment—does not perform the healing. It permits it. The most powerful interventions begin when you become an active participant in creating those conditions. That is a smaller claim than most health advice makes, and a more reliable one.

See Chapters 2 and 12

5. Health Is the Sum of Many Forces, Not Any Single One.

Health is rarely the result of a single factor. It is the accumulated result of nutrition, movement, sleep, light, stress, relationships, toxins, and experience acting together across years. No single intervention outweighs that sum. This is why the search for the one missing thing so reliably disappoints, and why the people who find it are usually the ones who stopped looking for it.

See Chapter 6

6. You Can't Get Better in the Environment That Made You Sick or Prevents You from Being Well.

Healing requires more than treatment. It requires that something change. If the conditions that produced the illness remain in place, the body has little reason to do anything different—and it will not. Even when those original conditions are gone, recovery can still be prevented if the body remains in an environment that cannot support repair. Change the conditions, and the biology changes with them.
See Chapter 6

7. Sunlight Is One of Biology's Strongest Signals.

For as long as there have been humans, sunlight has told the body what time it is. It anchors the master clock, and the clock governs hormone release, immune activity, digestion, and the overnight repair that determines whether you wake restored. Modern life has quietly removed this signal from most days. The body cannot keep accurate time on its own. It has to be calibrated by its environment.
See Chapter 7

8. Being Unwell Is Not a Problem Without a Solution. It Is a Puzzle That Can Be Solved with Patience and Time.

Symptoms are clues, not verdicts. The difficulty is rarely that no answer exists. It is that the answer sits upstream of where the symptom appears—and symptoms often appear where the hierarchy finally fails, not where the disruption first began. Look where it hurts and you will usually find the consequence. Look beneath it and you will find the cause.
See Chapters 3 and 7

9. Consistency Creates Conditions. Intensity Does Not.

The body reads repetition, not effort. A wake time held every morning teaches the clock more than any single perfect day. A recovery protocol

applied after every session—including the easy ones—teaches the system more than one heroic week. What discipline means in recovery is not pushing harder. It is doing the same small thing long enough that the body begins to expect it. Biology is not impressed by effort.
See Chapters 7 and 8

10. There Is a Universe Inside Us.
You are not a single organism. The microbes living in and on you help regulate digestion, immune signaling, metabolism, and the production of compounds your body depends on. They do not respond to intention. They respond to what you feed them, when you feed them, how you sleep, and whether the conditions around them are stable enough to support a community. Support them, and they support you.
See Chapter 6

A Note on the Science

The physiologic mechanisms described in this book—the autonomic regulatory hierarchy, the circadian clock and its peripheral clocks, mitochondrial signaling, the gut-immune-microbiome relationship, and the role of mechanical loading in structural repair—are grounded in peer-reviewed research across the fields of neuroscience, chronobiology, immunology, cellular metabolism, biomechanics, and exercise physiology. The Ettinger Foundation Protocol (EFP) framework integrates these established biologic principles into a clinical sequencing model that is, to my knowledge, original to this practice.

This book was written to make complex physiology understandable and clinically useful rather than to function as an academic textbook. A selected reference section follows for readers who wish to explore the scientific literature supporting the concepts presented throughout the book. The EFP Practitioner Manual expands substantially on these concepts, providing more detailed scientific discussion, additional mechanistic explanations, and an extensive reference library for clinicians and researchers who wish to examine the primary literature in greater depth.

Science continues to evolve. The principles presented in this book represent my best understanding of the available evidence and my clinical experience at the time of publication. As new research emerges, the EFP framework will continue to evolve with it.

To support that ongoing evolution, I have created www.thebookhealinginorder.com as the companion resource to this book. There, new research, clinical insights, and refinements to the EFP framework will be organized by phase of the regulatory hierarchy, allowing readers to follow developments in the science without having to search the medical literature themselves. My hope is that *Healing in Order* remains a living resource—

one that continues to grow as our understanding of human physiology grows, while preserving the biologic principles on which it was built.

The patient stories in this book are composite clinical narratives, as noted in the disclosure at the beginning of Chapter 1. They were created to illustrate real physiologic patterns observed across nearly four decades of clinical practice while protecting patient privacy. The physiologic patterns are real. The individuals they portray are not.

Readers are invited to visit www.thebookhealinginorder.com for updates on the research in this book, additional educational resources, and ongoing developments in the Ettinger Foundation Protocol (EFP) framework.

Selected References

Foundational Principles

Barrett, L. F., & Simmons, W. K. (2015). Interoceptive predictions in the brain. *Nature Reviews Neuroscience, 16*(7), 419–429.

Barrett, L. F., Quigley, K. S., & Hamilton, P. (2016). An active inference theory of allostasis and interoception in depression. *Philosophical Transactions of the Royal Society B: Biological Sciences, 371*(1708), 20160011.

Mattson, M. P. (2014). Superior pattern processing is the essence of the evolved human brain. *Frontiers in Neuroscience, 8*, Article 265.

Moseley, P., et al. (2021). Modelling the contribution of sensory processing, attention, and inhibitory control to schizophrenia using predictive processing. Frontiers in Human Neuroscience.

Sterling, P. (2012). Allostasis: A model of predictive regulation. *Physiology & Behavior, 106*(1), 5–15.

Sterling, P. (2018). Predictive regulation and human design. eLife, 7, e36133.

Theriault, J. E., Katsumi, Y., Reimann, H. M., Zhang, J., Deming, P., Dickerson, B. C., Quigley, K. S., & Barrett, L. F. (2025). It's not the thought that counts: Allostasis at the core of brain function. *Neuron, 113*(24), 4107–4133.

Turner, J. S. (2019). Homeostasis as a fundamental principle for a coherent theory of brains. *Philosophical Transactions of the Royal Society B: Biological Sciences, 374*(1774), 20180373.

Threat Assessment & Autonomic Regulation

Kavitha, N., Pal, P., Pal, G. K., Bharadwaj, B., & Nanda, N. (2024). Effects of slow breathing exercises on cardiac autonomic functions in anxiety disorder—A randomised control trial. *Annals of Neurosciences, 33*(3), 283–292.

Kim, T., Shin, M., & Woo, M. (2025). Autonomic nervous system activity in response to stress and cardiac coherence breathing exercise depending on body composition differences. *International Journal of Sport and Exercise Psychology, 23*(1), 40–56.

Levy, I., & Schiller, D. (2021). Neural computations of threat. *Trends in Cognitive Sciences, 25*(2), 151–171.

Nidhi, Singh, J. P., Antiwal, M., & Maurya, P. K. (2025). The therapeutic effects of Viparita Karani Mudra on non-communicable diseases. *International Research Journal of Ayurveda & Yoga, 8*(5), 69–72.

Pavlov, V. A., & Tracey, K. J. (2012). The vagus nerve and the inflammatory reflex—linking immunity and metabolism. *Nature Reviews Endocrinology, 8*(12), 743–754.

Porges, S. W. (2022). Polyvagal theory: A science of safety. *Frontiers in Integrative Neuroscience, 16*, Article 871227.

Circadian Biology & Sleep

Akgun, S. G., Gemici, B., Roddis, C., Bickerstaff, L., Bano Otalora, B., Milosavljevic, N., Brown, T. M., Lucas, R. J., & Didikoglu, A. (2026). Light exposure and sleep architecture in real-world settings. npj Biological Timing and Sleep, 3, Article 30.

Bass, J., & Takahashi, J. S. (2010). Circadian integration of metabolism and energetics. *Science, 330*(6009), 1349–1354.

Bellesi, M., Riedner, B. A., Garcia-Molina, G. N., Cirelli, C., & Tononi, G. (2014). Enhancement of sleep slow waves: Underlying mechanisms and practical consequences. *Frontiers in Systems Neuroscience, 8*, Article 208.

Biliński, K., Wiśniewski, K., Rafner, L., Witko, P., & Gaweł-Dąbrowska, D. (2026). Travel-induced circadian and microbiota disturbances: Implications for athlete health and performance: A narrative review. *Nutrients, 18*(10), 1523.

Brinkman, J. E., Reddy, V., & Sharma, S. (2023). Physiology of sleep. In StatPearls. StatPearls Publishing.

Chaix, A., & Panda, S. (2019). Timing tweaks exercise. *Nature Reviews Endocrinology, 15*(8), 440–441.

Gutierrez Lopez, D. E., Lashinger, L. M., Weinstock, G. M., & Bray, M. S. (2021). Circadian rhythms and the gut microbiome synchronize the host's metabolic response to diet. *Cell Metabolism, 33*(5), 873–887.

Hill, A. J., Eliopoulos, O., Emtage, J., Oikonomou, G., & Prober, D. A. (2026). Melatonin promotes sleep by suppressing responses to visual stimuli via MT1 receptors. *Current Biology, 36*(9), 2270–2284.e4.

Irwin, M. R. (2015). Why sleep is important for health: A psychoneuroimmunology perspective. *Annual Review of Psychology, 66*, 143–172.

Merrow, M. (2023). Circadian clocks: It's time for chronobiology. *PLOS Biology, 21*(11), e3002426.

O'Toole, C. K., et al. (2026). Sleep chart of biological ageing clocks in middle and late life. Nature.

Wang, M., Tsuno, Y., Peng, Y., Islam, M. T., Matsui, A., Maejima, T., & Mieda, M. (2026). Neuronal feedback loop of the suprachiasmatic nucleus generates robust circadian rhythms. *Nature Communications, 17*, Article 1505.

Zheng, B., Wang, L., Sun, S., Yuan, X., & Liang, Q. (2025). The molecular interplay between the gut microbiome and circadian rhythms: An integrated review. *Frontiers in Microbiology, 16*, 1712516.

Gut–Immune–Microbiome Physiology

Beurel, E. (2024). Stress in the microbiome-immune crosstalk. *Gut Microbes, 16*(1), 2327409.

Castells, M., et al. (2024). Mast cell activation syndrome: Current understanding and research needs. *Journal of Allergy and Clinical Immunology, 154*(2), 255–263.

Garcia, I., Kilic, F., Bryan, C.-A., Castro-Vildosola, J., Jonnalagadda, S. A., Kasturi, A., Tilly, J., Smith, J., Valentin, S., Moncayo, S., Hala, T., Klein, E., & Corbett, B. F. (2025). Social stress changes gut microbiome composition in male, female, and aggressor mice. *Brain, Behavior, & Immunity - Health, 50*, 101138.

Gwak, M.-G., & Chang, S.-Y. (2021). Gut-brain connection: Microbiome, gut barrier, and environmental sensors. *Immune Network, 21*(3), e20.

Environmental Physiology

Jimenez, M. P., DeVille, N. V., Elliott, E. G., Schiff, J. E., Wilt, G. E., Hart, J. E., & James, P. (2021). Associations between nature exposure and health: A review of the evidence. *International Journal of Environmental Research and Public Health, 18*(9), 4790.

Sudimac, S., Sale, V., & Kühn, S. (2022). How nature nurtures: Amygdala activity decreases as the result of a one-hour walk in nature. *Molecular Psychiatry, 27*(11), 4446–4452.

Clinical & Translational Medicine

Elsenbruch, S., & Enck, P. (2016). Psychobiological mechanisms in the pathophysiology of chronic visceral pain. *Schmerz, 30*(5), 407–411.

Hughes, J. R., John, E. R., Prichep, L. S., & Eastwood, M. R. (2008). The EEG in psychiatry: A practical approach. *Clinical EEG and Neuroscience, 39*(2), 109–116.

Mönnikes, H., Tebbe, J. J., Hildebrandt, M., Arck, P., Osmanoglou, E., Rose, M., Klapp, B., Wiedenmann, B., & Heymann-Mönnikes, I. (2001). Role of stress in functional gastrointestinal disorders: Evidence for stress-induced alterations in gastrointestinal motility and sensitivity. *Digestive Diseases, 19*(3), 201–211.

Structural Adaptation & Movement

Costamagna, D., Costelli, P., Sampaolesi, M., & Penna, F. (2015). Role of inflammation in muscle homeostasis and myogenesis. *Mediators of Inflammation, 2015*, 805172.

Guo, D. (2026). The regulatory effects of mechanical loading on cellular behavior during tendon–bone healing. *Materials & Design, 261*, 115364.

Plotkin, D., Coleman, M., Van Every, D., Maldonado, J., Oberlin, D., Israetel, M., Feather, J., Alto, A., Vigotsky, A. D., & Schoenfeld, B. J. (2022). Progressive overload without progressing load? The effects of load or repetition progression on muscular adaptations. *PeerJ, 10*, e14142.

Mitochondrial Biology & Cellular Energetics

Castro-Portuguez, R., & Sutphin, G. L. (2020). Kynurenine pathway, NAD+ synthesis, and mitochondrial function: Targeting tryptophan metabolism to promote longevity and healthspan. *Experimental Gerontology, 132*, Article 110841.

Goodpaster, B. H., & Sparks, L. M. (2017). Metabolic flexibility in health and disease. *Cell Metabolism, 25*(5), 1027–1036.

Jin, H., An, Y., Huang, J., Luo, T., & Wu, X. (2026). Pathophysiological mechanisms of post-exertional malaise: An integrative analysis based on the metabolism-immune-neuro interaction model. *Frontiers in Immunology, 17*, 1774310.

Kumar, P., Osahon, O., Sekhar, R. V., Sanborn, M., Sharma, D. R., Han, J., Freeman, M. L., & Jahoor, F. (2023). Supplementing glycine and N-acetylcysteine (GlyNAC) in older adults improves glutathione deficiency, oxidative stress, mitochondrial dysfunction, inflammation, physical function, and aging hallmarks: A randomized clinical trial. *The Journals of Gerontology: Series A, 78*(1), 75–89.

Mannino, P., Park, M., & Wang, M. C. (2026). Organellar insights in ageing and longevity. *Nature Cell Biology, 28*(5), 861–874.

Merz, K. E., & Thurmond, D. C. (2020). Role of skeletal muscle in insulin resistance and glucose uptake. *Comprehensive Physiology, 10*(3), 785–809.

Xu, X., Pang, Y., & Fan, X. (2025). Mitochondria in oxidative stress, inflammation and aging: From mechanisms to therapeutic advances. *Signal Transduction and Targeted Therapy, 10*, Article 190.

Acknowledgments

This book grew out of almost four decades of clinical practice and the thousands of patients who taught me, through the precision of their responses and the honesty of their experiences, what the body is actually doing when it appears to resist help. I am grateful to each of them—not for their suffering, but for their willingness to work with me through it, to trust a process that moved more slowly than they wanted, and to demonstrate, again and again, that the hierarchy holds.

I would not be the doctor I am today without the knowledge I have gained from reading the works of these brilliant and trailblazing mentors: Bruce Lipton, PhD; Robert Sapolsky, PhD; Rupert Sheldrake, PhD; Gerald Pollack, MD; Robert O. Becker, MD; Michael Crawford, PhD; Douglas Wallace, PhD; Dan Brule, Maynard Murray, MD; Stephanie Seneff, PhD; Alexander Wunsch, MD; Marcus Aurelius; and Epictetus.

About the Author

Marcus Ettinger, DC, is a clinician, educator, and researcher who has spent nearly four decades helping patients with complex chronic illness. A graduate of Southern California University of Health Sciences, formerly Los Angeles College of Chiropractic, he holds a Doctor of Chiropractic degree and a Bachelor of Science in Human Biology. Since entering private practice in Orange, California, in 1989, he has pursued an intensive study of evolutionary biology, microbiology, human biochemistry, clinical nutrition, diagnostic testing, and integrative approaches to healing. His work has taken him beyond the clinic as a lecturer, consultant, and practitioner serving patients and professionals around the world, from Ghana to Australia. In 2008, working under the name The Digestion Coach, he developed early clinical protocols addressing H. pylori and microbial biofilms—part of a growing clinical interest in how biofilm physiology contributes to persistent gastrointestinal and infectious conditions.

Decades of clinical observation eventually led Ettinger to a larger question: why do well-chosen treatments sometimes fail, produce only temporary improvement, or even make chronically ill patients worse? His answer became the Ettinger Foundation Protocol (EFP), a phase-based framework built around the principle that recovery depends not only on what is treated, but on whether the body is physiologically ready to respond. EFP organizes recovery according to biological sequence, beginning with foundational regulation and progressing through immune stability, circadian organization, cellular energy production, structural rebuilding, and long-term resilience. *Healing in Order* is the culmination of that work—a synthesis of nearly forty years of clinical experience, scientific study, and the recurring patterns observed in patients whose illnesses made far more sense once the order of healing was taken into account.

www.ingramcontent.com/pod-product-compliance
Lightning Source LLC
LaVergne TN
LVHW050812061126
851857LV00012B/774
* 9 7 9 8 9 9 7 5 1 3 4 2 9 *